STARLING'S LAW OF THE HEART REVISITED

edited by

HENK E.D.J. ter KEURS

Department of Medical Physiology, Medical Faculty,
The University of Calgary, Calgary, Alberta, Canada

MARK I.M. NOBLE

Consultant Physician, King Edward VII Hospital,
Midhurst, United Kingdom

KLUWER ACADEMIC PUBLISHERS
DORDRECHT / BOSTON / LONDON

Library of Congress Cataloging in Publication Data

Starling's law of the heart revisited / edited by Henk E.D.J. ter
  Keurs, Mark I.M. Noble.
      p.   cm. -- (Developments in cardiovascular medicine)
  Includes index.

    ISBN-13: 978-94-010-7084-3   e-ISBN-13: 978-94-009-1313-4
    DOI: 10.1007/978-94-009-1313-4

    1. Heart--Muscle. 2. Heart--Contraction.   I. Keurs, H. E. D. J.
  ter. II. Noble, Mark I. M. III. Series.
  QP113.2.S7 1988
  612'.17--dc19   88-12692
                                                     CIP

Published by Kluwer Academic Publishers,
P.O. Box 17, 3300 AA Dordrecht, The Netherlands.

Kluwer Academic Publishers incorporates
the publishing programmes of
D. Reidel, Martinus Nijhoff, Dr W. Junk and MTP Press.

Sold and distributed in the U.S.A. and Canada
by Kluwer Academic Publishers,
101 Philip Drive, Norwell, MA 02061, U.S.A.

In all other countries, sold and distributed
by Kluwer Academic Publishers,
P.O. Box 322, 3300 AH Dordrecht, The Netherlands.

Table of Contents

The greater the length of the fibre, and therefore the greater amount of surface of its longitudinal contractile elements at the moment when it begins to contract, the greater will be the energy in the form of contractile stress set up in its contraction, and the more extensive will be the chemical changes involved. This relation between the length of the heart fibre and its power of contraction I have called "the law of the heart."

E.H. Starling (1920)
On the circulatory changes associated with exercise
J. Roy. Army Med. Corps 34: 258–272

List of Major Contributors

Dr. D.G. Allen, Department of Physiology, University College of London, London, Gower Street, London WC1E-6BT, United Kingdom

Dr. T. Arts, Biomedical Centre, University of Limburg, 6200 MD Maastricht, The Netherlands

Dr. G. Elzinga, Laboratory for Physiology, Free University of Amsterdam, 1081 BT Amsterdam, The Netherlands

Dr. P.R. Housmans, Department of Anesthesiology, Mayo Foundation, Rochester, MN 55905, U.S.A.

Dr. T. Iwazumi, Department of Medical Physiology, Health Science Centre, University of Calgary, Calgary, Alberta, Canada T2N-4N1

Dr. J.C. Kentish, Department of Physiology, University College of London, Gower Street, London WC1E-6BT, United Kingdom

Dr. J.W. Krueger, Albert Einstein College of Medicine, Bronx, New York, NY 10461, U.S.A.

Dr. M.I.M. Noble, King Edward VII Hospital, Midhurst, West Sussex GU29-0BL, United Kingdom

Dr. K. Sagawa, Department of Biomedical Engineering, Johns Hopkins University Medical School, Baltimore, MD 21205, U.S.A.

Dr. H.E.D.J. ter Keurs, Department of Medical Physiology, Faculty of Medicine, Health Science Centre, University of Calgary, Calgary, Alberta, Canada T2N-4N1

Introduction

H.E.D.J. TER KEURS & M.I.M. NOBLE

The "Starling's Law of the Heart" and "The Frank-Starling Mechanism" have long been the cornerstone of cardiac mechanical physiology. It is often forgotten that Frank and Starling carried out fundamentally different experiments. Frank[1] measured the isovolumic pressure developed by frog heart at different volumes. He therefore discovered the pressure-volume-volume relationship which depends directly on the force-length relationship of the sarcomeres. Starling[2,3] studied cardiac shortening as manifest by cardiac output and its relationship to end-diastolic conditions as manifest by right atrial pressure. Thus he was studying the ability of cardiac muscle to shorten more at a given load from a greater initial length. Starling in the promulgations of his law[4] implied a common mechanism for these two phenomena and spoke of the "energy liberated" being a function of initial muscle fiber length. However, there has been much confusion about the interrelationship between the two different aspects studied by Frank and Starling.

The 1960s saw the era of isolated cardiac muscle mechanics, beginning with the paper of Abbott and Mommaerts.[5] Whole muscle length-tension relations were equated with sarcomere-length-tension relations by fixation of muscle at a particular point on the curve and determination of sarcomere length by electronmicroscopy.[6] When the Ciba Symposium "Physiological Basis of Starling's Law of the Heart" was held in 1973 (published 1974),[7] the field was at a very exciting stage as the first attempts at instantaneous sarcomere length, measured during the experiment on the living muscle, were reported. In the decade since that publication, definitive data collected with these methods have appeared.[8,9] These advances are summarized and brought up to date in the present volume.

Chapter 1 of the Ciba Symposium[7] contained considerable discussion on the mechanism of the increased mechanical performance of cardiac muscle when stretched. These were summarized by Jewell[10], who predicted that variations in activation of the myofilaments by calcium ions would probably prove to be the mechanism. Nevertheless, Jewell was the first to disprove this

H.E.D.J. ter Keurs and M.I.M. Noble (eds), Starling's Law of the Heart Revisited. ISBN 978-94-010-7084-3
© 1988, Kluwer Academic Publishers, Dordrecht

idea. In his paper with Hibberd,[11] it was shown that in chemically skinned cardiac muscle, a shift in the relationship of force to calcium ion concentration was found. This was confirmed in much greater detail by Kentish et al.[12] whose data also explain the change in shape of sarcomere length-force curves with increasing extracellular Ca^{2+} in intact fibres. These new findings are summarized and brought up to date in Chapter 4; those factors other than a change in sensitivity of the myofilaments to Ca^{2+} which may still be considered to contribute are explained. Furthermore, disproof of Jewell's hypothesis is given by (1) the lack of effect of instantaneous length changes on intracellular Ca^{2+} (Chapter 3); (2) the failure of changes in length to change calcium induced calcium release from the sarcoplasmic reticulum (Chapter 1); and (3) the presence of a positive sarcomere length-tension curve at constant Ca^{2+} in isolated myofibrils (Chapter 2). We are most grateful to Dr. A. Fabiato for carrying out further experiments on this point with his latest methods and for allowing us to publish his negative results. The new methods of instantaneous sarcomere length measurement have produced a lower yield of new information on shortening behavior of cardiac muscle. Effects of shortening per se on contractile properties continue to be perplexing (Chapters 4 and 5). Velocity of sarcomere shortening at zero load (V_o, V_{max}) has been well characterized in rat muscle (Chapter 6) but not in other species.

The development of understanding of the Frank and Starling phenomena in the intact heart has attracted less attention, both prior to and since the 1973 Ciba Symposium.[7] The major contributions have been: (1) the development of the pressure-volume diagram of the left ventricle as the best means for understanding, integrating, and interpreting cardiac muscle length-tension and length shortening characteristics (Chapters 7, 10); (2) greater accuracy in the study of the geometric factors relating muscle fibres to whole heart function (Chapter 8); and (3) the approach to the whole subject from engineering criteria for assessment of the heart as a pump (Chapter 9).

The idea of collecting these contributions into a book arose from a widespread feeling that there was a need to update the classic book from the Ciba Symposia 1973. This feeling manifested itself in a series of meetings in recent years. The Cardiac Muscle Research Group in the United Kingdom held a meeting at Bath in 1985 entitled "Frank and Starling Revisited" followed by an indepth small Symposium at Midhurst for the speakers. These meetings were preceded and followed by Symposia of the Physiological Society at St. Andrews and Leiden. None of these meetings were published apart from the abstracts of the CMRG.[13] We have therefore tried to obtain contributions to a new book that would be an appropriate update to the Ciba publication. We are very grateful to those contributors to the meeting who did not feel able to submit Chapters to the present publication. We would particularly like to mention Dr. Brian Jewell, Chairman of the CMRG meeting at Bath and leader and instigator of studies of the subject over the years, Dr. A. Guz, his co-Chairman and also Chairman of the Ciba Symposium, 1973, and Dr. D.J. Miller[18] and to Dr. Denis Noble, Chairman of the Leiden Symposium. Important contributions not included here were those of Matsubara, Maughan and Yagi[14] and of Lloyd Hefner.[15]

The discussions during these meetings foreboded a considerable number of future developments, both to address important unanswered questions and to resolve some points of disagreement between participants, e.g.: (1) when muscle length is increased there is an immediate fast response of force followed by a more slowly developing further force increase which is accompanied by an increase in calcium release. This phenomenon was found by the groups of Allen, Nichols and Hefner but not by those of Krueger, Sagawa or Noble. "Why are the results of these groups different" (2) Miller found hysteresis in the calcium versus tension relationship of chemically "skinned" cardiac muscle[18] whereas Kentish and ter Keurs did not. "Which result is correct" Both of these controversies are of considerable importance, and have a potentially large effect on our present ideas of how the heart behaves within the pressure-volume diagram.

At the time of writing, the force-sarcomere length relationship of cardiac muscle appears to be mainly attributable to a length dependent change in the sensitivity of the contractile proteins to calcium.[16,17] Some evidence points to this being a change in the affinity of troponin for Ca^{2+} (Chapters 1, 6). Mechanical data suggests cooperativity between force generation and Ca^{2+} binding. We expect that the answer to the question whether this mechanism determines the force-sarcomere length relation may emerge in the next years.

The role of restoring forces in the force-sarcomere length relationship is postulated at present on the basis of indirect findings and more by exclusion than by direct evidence (Chapter 1). Improved measurement techniques (Chapter 2) may be expected to yield the relevant data on the magnitude of restoring forces as a function of sarcomere length in the near future.

Little is known about the effects of activation and sarcomere length on the relation between force and velocity. We anticipate that the combination of studies of sarcomere dynamics with the use of caged compounds in the analysis of the kinetics of myofibrillar ATP hydrolysis will reveal exciting insights into the molecular mechanism of cardiac contraction in the next decade.

To what extent does the behavior of intact rat heart muscle (Chapter 1) represent heart muscle in general and human heart muscle in particular. This question follows from the higher level of activation found in rat compared to other mammalia. We should therefore expect the modern techniques summarized in these pages to be extended to such species as rabbit, cat, dog and man. It also has been shown that the end-systolic pressure volume relation is non linear (Chapter 7). Further studies of the independence of this relation on diastolic and systolic conditions are still required. For example, the deactivating effect of shortening has been confirmed in isolated muscle (Chapter 6) but it is not clear whether this accounts for differences between the isovolumic and end-systolic pressure-volume relationships of the intact heart (Chapter 7) or whether the latter are merely a manifestation of the limitations of the duration of systole (Chapter 10).

The analysis of Chapter 8 suggests the exciting possibility that we can drop complex geometric models of the ventricles when considering force-sarcomere length relationships in the intact heart. We may be able to consider merely a long one-dimensional muscle bundle, wrapped around the cavity, in which only the cavity volume and mass of muscle contribute to the translation of force-sarcomere length to pressure-volume. On the other hand, an increasing body of evidence suggests that the pericardium[19] exerts a constraining effect on the heart under conditions in which it previously has been considered to be of little relevance. Further information regarding the effect of the pericardium on coupling of the function of the cardiac compartments will emerge with new techniques to assess its properties.

Finally, we anticipate an answer in the next decade to the question posed by the finding that the working point of the heart corresponds to maximum power transfer from heart to arterial system (Chapter 9). Does this result solely from the pressure-volume diagram (Chapter 10) which will tend to always move the heart towards a maximum pressure-volume loop or must one invoke mechanisms other than the Frank and Starling phenomena The quest for a mechanism that is utilized by the organism to maximize the transfer of power from the heart to the vascular system will provide insight in the regulation of cardiac growth as the adaptive mechanism, which is superimposed on the neurohumoral and length-dependent regulation of cardiac function as was discussed by Starling.[20]

References

1. Frank O (1885). Zur Dynamik des Heizmuskels, Zeitschrift fur Biologie 32:370–447, translated by Chapman CB and Wasserman E (1959). Am Heart J 58: 282–317, 467–478.
2. Patterson SW, Piper H and Starling EH (1914). The regulation of the heart beat. J Physiol 48: 465–513.
3. Patterson SW and Starling EH (1914). On the mechanical factors which determine the output of the ventricles. J Physiol 48: 357–379.
4. Starling EH (1918). The Linacre Lecture on the Law of the Heart, Jougmans, Green and Co, London.
5. Abbott BC and Mommeart WFHM (1959). A study of inotropic mechanisms in the papillary muscle preparation. J Gen Physiol 42: 533–551.

6. Sonnenblick EH and Skelton CL (1974). Reconsideration of the ultra-structural basis of cardiac length-tension relations. Circ Res 35: 517–526.
7. Ciba Foundation Symposium (1974): The PHysiological Basis of Starling's Law of the Heart. Elsevier: Excerpta Medica: North Holland, Amsterdam.
8. ter Keurs HEDJ, Rijnsburger WH, van Heunigen R and Nagelsmit MJ (1980). Tension development and sarcomere length in rat cardiac trabeculae. Evidence of length-dependent activation. Circ Res 46: 703–714.
9. Daniels M, Noble MIM, ter Keurs HEDJ and Wohlfart B (1984). Velocity of sarcomere shortening in rat cardiac muscle: relationship to force sarcomere length, calcium and time. J Physiol 355: 367–381.
10. Jewell BR (1977). A re-examination of the influence of muscle length on myocardial performance. Circ Res 40: 221–230.
11. Hibberd MG and Jewell BR (1982). Calcium- and length-dependent force production in rat ventricular muscle. J Physiol 329: 527–540.
12. Kentish JC, ter Keurs HEDJ, Ricciardi L, Bucx JJJ and Noble MIM (1986). Comparison between the sarcomere length-force relations of intact and skinned trabeculae from rat right ventricle. Circ Res 58: 755–768.
13. Abstracts of symposium organized by the Cardiac Muscle Research Group (1985). Cardiovasc Res 19: 513–524.
14. Matsubara I, Maughan DW and Yagi N (1985). An X-ray diffraction study of chemically skinned cardiac muscle. Cardiovasc Res 19: 514.
15. Reeves RC, Reeves DNS, Walker AA and Hefner LL (1985). The fast and slow components of the force-length curve in cardiac muscle. Cardiovasc Res 19: 520.
16. Housmans PK, Lee NK and Blinks JR (1983a). Active cellular calcium transient in mammalian heart muscle. Science 221: 159–161.
17. Housmans PK, Lee NK and Blinks JR (1983b). History of loading in preceding contractions influences intracellular calcium transients in cat papillary muscle. Fed Proc 42: 573.
18. Harrison SM, Lamont C and Miller DJ (1985). Hysteresis in the Ca vs. tension relationship of chemically "skinned" cardiac muscle. J Physiol 364: 91P.
19. Tyberg JV, Taichman GC, Smith ER, Douglas NWS, Smiseth OA, and Keon WJ (1986). The relationship between pericardial pressure and right atrial pressure: an intraoperative study. Circulation 73: 428–432.
20. Starling EH (1919). On the circulatory changes associated with exercise. Lecture given at the Army Medical College 1919. In "Starling on the Heart". CB Chapman, JH Mitchell, Dawsons of Pall Mall, London.

1. The Contribution of Myofibrillar Properties to the Sarcomere Length–Force Relationship of Cardiac Muscle

J.C. KENTISH, H.E.D.J. TER KEURS & D.G. ALLEN

Department of Physiology, University College London, London, U.K.; Department of Medicine & Medical Physiology, The University of Calgary, Health Sciences Centre, Alberta, Canada

Abstract

The relationship between sarcomere length and active force was explored in detergent skinned cardiac trabeculae. This skinning technique removes any contribution of variable calcium release, the myofibrillar Ca^{2+} being that of the activating solution. Under these circumstances active force increases with sarcomere length from 1.6 μm to 2.3 μm, perhaps as much as in intact fibres. In order to test the possibility that this was due to a change in number of active myosin sites an indirect method of assessing myosin ATPase activity was used, namely measurement of the time required to produce rigor in the absence of ATP and PCr.

The results were essentially negative. The different shapes of the force–SL curves (concave to the force axis at low $[Ca^{2+}]$, convex at high $[Ca^{2+}]$) suggested a change in sensitivity of the contractile proteins to $[Ca^{2+}]$. This was confirmed by showing that the force versus $[Ca^{2+}]$ relationships shifted to the left with increasing sarcomere length. To test whether this was due to a change in the affinity of troponin for Ca^{2+}, we rapidly shortened aequorin loaded fibres. This caused an emission of light indicating release of Ca^{2+} from troponin to cause the light emitting reaction between Ca^{2+} and aequorin and confirming the likelihood that the sarcomere shortening reduced the affinity of troponin for Ca^{2+}. That this change might be caused by a change in spacing of the myofilament lattice appears disproved by experiments in which lattice spacing was varied with different dextran solutions. Thus the principle finding of this study is that most or all of the ascending limb of the force–SL curve of heart muscle can be accounted for by mechanisms other than changes in calcium release; such changes in calcium release appear less important than formerly according to the most recent results of Fabiato also reported here in preliminary form (Appendix).

H.E.D.J. ter Keurs and M.I.M. Noble (eds), Starling's Law of the Heart Revisited. ISBN 978-94-010-7084-3
© 1988, Kluwer Academic Publishers, Dordrecht

Introduction

The range of sarcomere lengths (SL) found in working cardiac muscle is narrow, from about 1.6 μm to about 2.3 μm. Nevertheless, over this limited range active force development varies from a maximum at 2.3 μm to zero at 1.6 μm i.e. the SL–force relationship is very steep (e.g. Fig. 1A). This sensitivity of force to SL is an essential component of the Frank-Starling mechanism, by which stroke volume is influenced by the diastolic filling of the heart. In contrast to cardiac muscle, in tetanized skeletal fibers developed force varies by about 20% over the same SL range of 1.6–2.3 μm,[1] suggesting that the force production of striated muscle myofibrils is rather insensitive to SL when the myofibrils are fully activated with Ca^{2+}. In the studies described here, we have tried to establish the factors responsible for the cardiac SL–force relationship and to determine why it is that force production falls so markedly as the SL is decreased in cardiac muscle. There are two main possible explanations for the decrease in force at shorter SL: (i) a decrease in the Ca^{2+} transient, causing less activation of the myofibrils, or (ii) a decrease in the force generated by the myofibrils at a given $[Ca^{2+}]$. We have attempted to distinguish these possibilities by using skinned cardiac fibers, in which the cell membranes have been destroyed so that the ionic environment of the myofibrils can be controlled by the solution bathing the muscle. This allows the $[Ca^{2+}]$ to be held constant at predetermined levels so that factor (i) above can be eliminated; any length-dependent properties of the skinned muscle preparation can then be ascribed to factor (ii). In this way it is possible to assess the contribution of myofibrillar properties to the SL–force relationship of intact (unskinned) cardiac muscle.

Sarcomere length–force relationships in intact and skinned muscles

To provide a comparison between intact and skinned muscles, we determined the SL–force relationships in the same muscles (rat ventricular trabeculae) before and after the muscles were skinned.[2] It was of particular interest to establish the SL–force relationships in the skinned muscles at *submaximal* concentrations of Ca^{2+}, because these are the concentrations found in intact cardiac muscle during the twitch.[3] SL was measured continuously with a laser diffraction system.[4] This was found to be essential, as the compliant damaged ends of the muscles allowed shortening of the central sarcomeres by 10%–20% during contraction, even though the muscle contraction was isometric. This internal shortening occurred both in the intact muscle[5] and in the skinned muscles. Thus the SL of the central sarcomeres during contraction was considerably less than in the relaxed muscle.

Fig. 1 shows the mean results from intact muscles (Fig. 1A) and from skinned muscles (Fig. 1B). For the intact muscles, muscle length was altered from the control length for 4 beats and active force and SL were measured at the instant of peak force in the 4th beat. The muscle was then returned to the control length for at least 6 beats. Force in the intact muscle was zero at SL = 1.55 μm; above this SL, force rose steeply in 1.5 mM Ca^{2+} and less steeply at 0.3 mM Ca^{2+}. The SL–force relationships were curved in different directions at the two Ca^{2+} concentrations. Thus, as noted previously[4] there is not a single SL–force relationship; rather its shape and slope depend upon the degree of Ca^{2+}-activation of the muscle. This indicates that length must be affecting the degree of Ca^{2+}-activation of the myofibrils in the muscle.

It should be noted that the protocol described above to determine the SL–force relationship allowed no time for the slow changes in active force that are seen 10–100 beats after the change to a new muscle length.[6] These slow changes cause the "steady-state" SL–force relationship to be even steeper than the "immediate" relationship of Fig. 1A (see Jewell[7]). There is good evidence that these slow changes are due to alterations in the amount of Ca^{2+} supplied to the myofibrils during the twitch.[8]

Once the relationship was determined in the intact trabecula, the muscle was skinned with Triton X-100 for 30 min.[9] The skinned muscles were bathed in an artificial cytosol (see legend to Fig. 1B), with the $[Ca^{2+}]$ set at the desired level by CaEGTA buffers. The muscle was bathed in a particular $[Ca^{2+}]$ and the SL–force relationship determined by briefly stretching the muscle to different lengths and measuring SL and active force. Force was zero at SL 1.5–1.7 μm (Fig. 1B). At longer SL, the steepness of the force–SL relationships depended upon the $[Ca^{2+}]$, and there was the same change of curvature with increasing $[Ca^{2+}]$ as was seen in the intact muscle. Indeed, the relationships for the skinned muscle at moderate level of Ca^{2+}-activation (4.3 μM and 8.9 μM Ca^{2+}) resembled those for the same muscle prior to skinning. Each curve for the skinned muscle was determined at constant $[Ca^{2+}]$, so the force–SL relationships of Fig. 1B must reflect the properties of the myofibrils (and connective tissue – see below) rather than of the Ca^{2+} supply to the myofibrils. From the similarity between the curves for the intact and skinned muscles, we may conclude that a large part of the SL–force relationship in the intact muscle may be due to the Ca^{2+}- and SL-dependent properties of the cardiac myofibrils.

All the SL–force relationships for the intact muscle, and those for the skinned muscles at submaximal $[Ca^{2+}]$ (below 50 μM Ca^{2+}) converged to zero force at a SL of 1.6 μm or so. As this SL is close to the length of the myosin filaments (1.55 μm), it seems likely that the loss of force at this SL was a result of the myosin filaments from adjacent sarcomeres reaching the Z-band and resisting further shortening of the sarcomeres. In effect, such

4

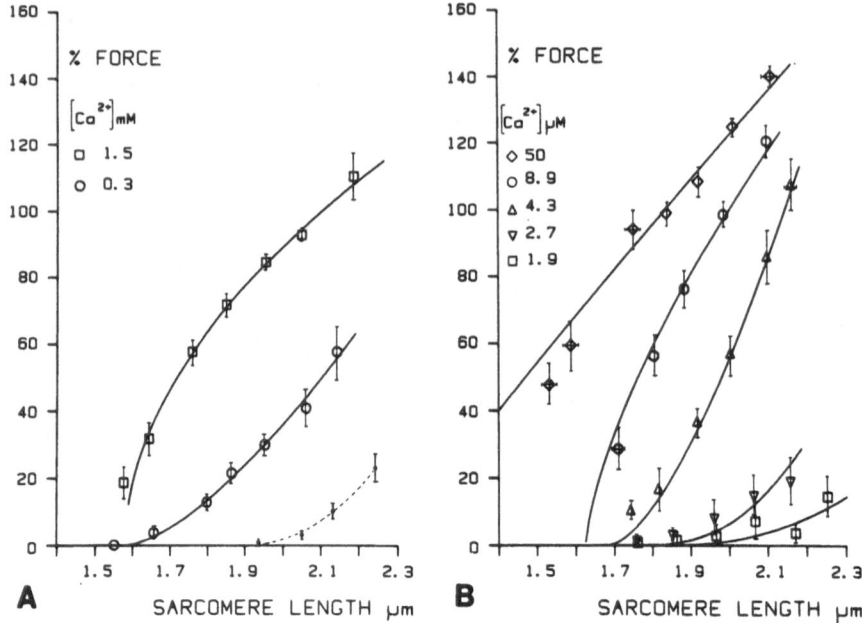

Fig. 1. Relationship between force production and sarcomere length (SL) in six rat trabeculae before and after skinning. SL was averaged in 0.1 μm bins. *A.* Active force (open symbols) in intact trabeculae bathed in Tyrode's solution with 1.5 mM or 0.3 mM extracellular Ca^{2+}. The passive force–SL relationship is also shown (dashed line). Points show mean ± S.E.. Stimulation rate 0.2 Hz. *B.* Active force in the same trabeculae after they had been skinned. $[Ca^{2+}]$ was set at the values shown with Ca:EGTA buffers. Solutions also contained (in mM): 140 K^+, 30 Na^+, 3 Mg^{2+}, 20 BES, 100 propionate, 5 $MgATP^2$), 10 phosphocreatine (PCr), 1 dithiothreitol, 25 ug/ml creatine kinase; pH 7.0. Below 1.9 μM Ca^{2+} no active force was produced (results not shown). For both the intact and skinned muscles "active force" was calculated as the total force minus the passive force at the same SL. Temperature 22°C–25°C throughout. (From Kentish et al.[2], with permission).

myofilament interactions would produce a strong force (restoring force or internal load) that acted against the force generated by the active cross-bridges, so decreasing the net force developed by the muscle.

The SL–force relationship at full Ca^{2+}-activation of the myofibrils (at 50 μM Ca^{2+} and above) differed from the results at lower levels of activation in that force production at SL = 1.6 μm was not zero but was about 40% of the force at SL = 2.2 μm. However, even this modest reduction of force at 1.6 μm was considerably greater than that found by Fabiato & Fabiato[10] with single skinned cardiac cells at maximal activation: in single cells, force at 1.6 μm was only 15% lower than that at 2.2 μm. It could be that the properties of the myofibrils are different in trabeculae and in single cells. However, a more likely explanation for the discrepancy is that in the trabeculae at shorter SL, there is an additional restoring force that opposes sarcomere shortening and so reduces the measured force generation. As this internal load seems to be present in skinned trabeculae (a multicellular preparation) but not in the skinned single cells used by Fabiato & Fabiato, it may be due to extracellular connective tissue or to intercellular connections[11] which are lacking in the single cells. It is possible that the element which is responsible for this restoring force in trabeculae and which must be acting in parallel with the sarcomeres, is the same parallel elastic element that prevents stretch of the sarcomeres above 2.3 μm in these preparations; in other words, it may oppose SL changes both above and below the slack length of the myofibrils (about 1.95 μm).

Further evidence for a restoring force during maximal Ca^{2+}-activation in skinned trabeculae at short sarcomere lengths

In 1966, Gordon, Huxley & Julian[1] pointed out that the decrease in force at SL below the optimum in skeletal fibers could be due to a decrease in the number of actively-cycling crossbridges or to an increase in internal load. The fact that the fall of force at short SL is small in single skinned cells[10] suggests that the decrease in force in the skinned trabeculae is not likely to be due entirely to a decrease in the number of active crossbridges (if we assume that the properties of myofibrils in single cells and in trabeculae are similar). An internal load at shorter SL in the trabeculae is also consistent with the finding that the maximum velocity of unloaded shortening in intact muscle decreases as SL is reduced below 1.9 μm.[12] A more direct way to distinguish between the two possibilities suggested by Gordon, Huxley & Julian[1] is to determine the ATPase activity at different sarcomere lengths, in order to measure the number of cycling crossbridges.

This has been done in skinned trabeculae (from rat and ferret hearts) by an indirect method, which makes use of the following observation: if a Ca^{2+}-activated skinned muscle is put into oil so that ATP and phosphocreatine (PCr) can no longer be supplied by the external bathing solution, the continuing actomyosin ATPase activity will cause the [ATP] and [PCr] inside the muscle to fall and eventually the muscle will go into rigor. The time course of these changes in force reflects the ATPase activity in the muscle and therefore can be used as an approximate measure of the ATPase activity. Fig. 2A shows what happens when a Ca^{2+}-activated skinned muscle is put into mineral oil. The force decreases initially, probably as a result of the accumulation of Pi, which inhibits force production,[13] but then increases to reach a plateau as the muscle goes into rigor. Rigor force in the presence of Ca^{2+} is about 50% greater than maximum Ca^{2+}-regulated force (Kentish, unpublished observations; cf. Kawai & Brandt[14]). (The initial rate of force decline in oil can also be used as a measure of Pi production and thus of the ATPase activity; the

6

same conclusions are obtained as if the overall timecourse is used.) If the [Ca²⁺] is only enough to give 60% of maximum force (Fig. 2A), the timecourse is prolonged by about 60%, indicating that the ATPase activity is reduced by about this amount. However if the force production is again reduced by 60%, but this time by decreasing muscle length at saturating [Ca²⁺], a different result is obtained (Fig. 2B). The time-course is only slightly prolonged (by about 5%) by this manoeuvre. This suggests that the decrease in muscle length causes only a small reduction in ATPase activity, whereas force is reduced to a much greater extent. Therefore a fall in the number of active crossbridges can account for only a small part of the fall of

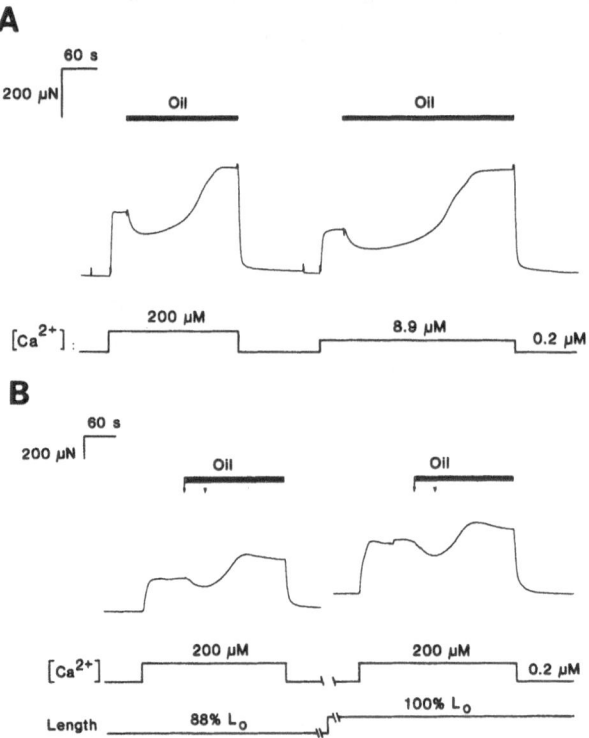

Fig. 2. Effect of placing Ca^{2+}-activated skinned trabeculae from ferret in oil to remove the external source of ATP and PCr. A. Influence of $[Ca^{2+}]$. The muscle was first activated in 200 μM or 8.9 μM Ca^{2+} with 5 mM MgATP + 10 mM PCr before transfer into water)saturated mineral oil (for the period shown by the solid bars). The muscle was then returned to relaxing solution (0.2 μM Ca^{2+}). B. Influence of muscle length. Muscle length is given as a % of the optimal length for force production (Lo). The muscle was activated in each case with the saturating $[Ca^{2+}]$ of 200 μM. The arrows show the time between the application of oil and the point of minimum force in oil. It was found that the fall of force in oil and the timecourse of rigor formation was about 5% slower at the shorter muscle length although the Ca^{2+}-regulated force was reduced by 40%. Different muscle from that in trace A. Similar results were found in two other experiments. (Kentish, unpublished observations.)

force. From this it seems likely that the reduced force at short muscle lengths in skinned trabeculae is due chiefly to an increased restoring force. This conclusion is also supported by the observation that maximum Ca^{2+}-activated force and rigor force were reduced by the same absolute amount at the shorter muscle length (Fig. 2B), even though the decrease in rigor force cannot have been due to a reduced number of active crossbridges. These results emphasize the importance of internal loads in influencing force development at maximal Ca^{2+}, although the conclusions should be treated with caution until these preliminary experiments are repeated with a more direct measure of ATPase activity.

SL-dependent changes in the sensitivity of myofibrils to Ca^{2+}

In the preceding section it was argued that restoring forces could account for a large part of the SL–force relationship in skinned trabeculae at maximal $[Ca^{2+}]$. However, at least one other factor must contribute at submaximal $[Ca^{2+}]$, for the relationships at submaximal Ca^{2+} showed changes in slope, and were steeper in places than at maximal Ca^{2+} (Fig. 1B); this is not as would be expected if shortening the muscle merely decreased maximum force and submaximal force in proportion. One factor is that there was an increase in Ca^{2+}-sensitivity of the myofibrils as the SL was raised. This can be seen more clearly if the curves in Fig. 1B are replotted to show the force–$[Ca^{2+}]$ relationships at selected sarcomere lengths (Fig. 3). Each increase in SL not only increased the maximum force but also shifted the force–$[Ca^{2+}]$ relationships to lower $[Ca^{2+}]$, i.e. the Ca^{2+}-sensitivity of the myofibrils was increased. In addition, the slope of the force–$[Ca^{2+}]$ relationship was greater at the longer SL. These changes occurred over the entire range of SL found in intact cardiac muscle (1.6–2.3 μm). This confirms and extends previous work by Fabiato[15] and Hibberd & Jewell.[16] This effect makes an important contribution to the steepness of the SL–force relationship in the skinned muscles at submaximal $[Ca^{2+}]$ (Fig. 1B) and, by implication, in the intact muscles, too.

What causes the increase in Ca^{2+}-sensitivity at longer sarcomere lengths

Changes in Ca^{2+}-sensitivity with SL such as those shown in Fig. 3 have now been observed in a variety of preparations from both cardiac muscle and skeletal muscle (for review, see Allen & Kentish[17]) although the precise mechanism of this effect remains unclear. One possible explanation is that the affinity of troponin for Ca^{2+} increases with SL. Alternatively the Ca^{2+}-

affinity of troponin may not be sensitive to SL, in which case we must assume that the SL-dependence of Ca^{2+}-sensitivity arises from a step in the activation sequence that occurs after the binding of Ca^{2+} to troponin. An attempt was made to distinguish between these two possibilities by using the following approach.[18] Detergent-skinned muscles (from ferret or rat ventricles) were activated with a $[Ca^{2+}]$ that gave about 80% of maximum force and were then released suddenly to decrease muscle length and thus decrease SL. If the Ca^{2+}-affinity of troponin were dependent upon SL, we would expect the amount of Ca^{2+} bound to troponin to be less at the shorter SL and some Ca^{2+} would be released from the myofibrils. Alternatively, if Ca^{2+}-affinity were insensitive to SL, no Ca^{2+} would be released. The skinned trabeculae were loaded with the photoprotein aequorin to detect any release of Ca^{2+} from the myofibrils. The $[Ca^{2+}]$ was very lightly buffered with 100 μM EGTA for these experiments. Fig. 4 shows the response to shortening in a muscle that had been loaded with aequorin for 10 min (at <0.1 μM Ca^{2+}) and then activated in 15 μM Ca^{2+}. The decrease in muscle length caused an increase in the light emitted from aequorin, indicating that the $[Ca^{2+}]$ inside the muscle had increased (from 15 μM to 16 μM in this case). When the muscle was restretched to the control length, force rose and light emission fell to their previous levels. Because all the Ca^{2+}-sequestering organelles had been destroyed by the detergent, the Ca^{2+} released at the shorter muscle length must have come from the myofibrils. This Ca^{2+} was almost certainly released from troponin. These results support the idea that the Ca^{2+}-affinity of troponin decreases with decreasing SL. However, the unknown distribution of aequorin in the muscles makes it difficult to assess quantitatively the change in Ca^{2+} binding to troponin. Therefore we do not know whether the decrease in Ca^{2+}-affinity of troponin (Fig. 4) is sufficient to account for the observed SL-dependence of myofibrillar Ca^{2+}-sensitivity (Fig. 3).

It is of interest to compare the time-courses of length, force and light after the muscle was restretched (Fig. 4). Although muscle length was increased within 10 ms, force took about 1 s to reach a steady level; this slow force response to stretch is a characteristic of cardiac, and some other, muscles[19] and is probably due to a slow increase in the number of myosin crossbridges attached to actin. Light decreased with the same slow time-course as the increase in force, but this was very different from the sudden change in muscle length. Thus it may be that the Ca^{2+}-affinity of troponin is more closely related to force development than to SL itself. One way to assimilate these data is by supposing that the Ca^{2+}-affinity of troponin is determined by crossbridge attachment; there is some evidence for this, at least for rigor attachment of crossbridges in skeletal muscle.[20] On this basis, the slow attachment of crossbridges after restretch of the muscle causes not only increased force production but also an increase in the Ca^{2+}-affinity of

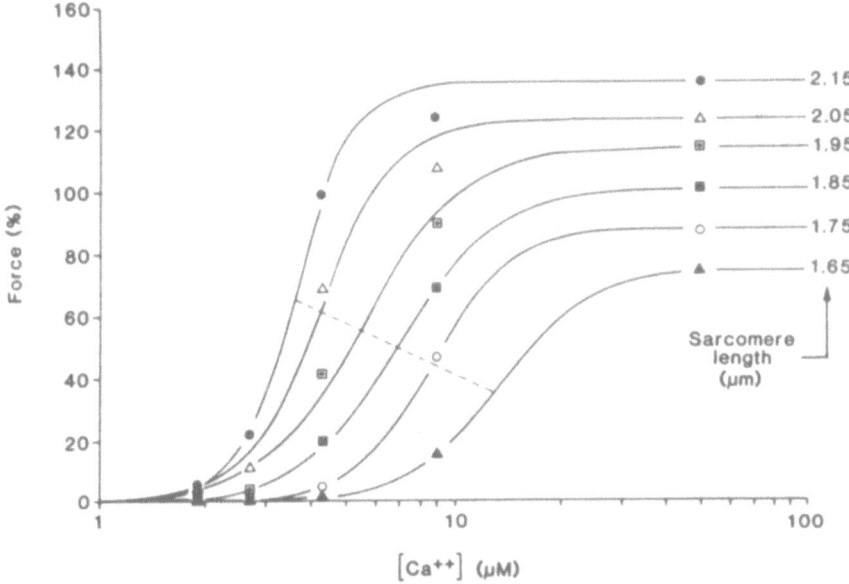

Fig. 3. Relationship between active force and $[Ca^{2+}]$ in skinned muscles at various SL (given in μm next to the appropriate curves). Data obtained by replotting the curves of Fig. 1B. The solid lines are best-fits to the modified Hill equation:

$$Force = Maximum\ force \times [Ca^{2+}]^n / (K + [Ca^{2+}]^n)$$

The dashed line joins the points corresponding to half)maximal activation for each curve. It can be seen that increasing the SL raises both maximum force production and the Ca^{2+}-sensitivity of the myofibrils. (Kentish et al.[2])

troponin, which results in a fall of $[Ca^{2+}]$ inside the muscle and a fall of light. If this is so, it is possible that a part, at least, of the SL-dependence of myofibrillar Ca^{2+}-sensitivity (Fig. 3) is mediated by crossbridge attachment: the SL may determine the maximum number of crossbridges that can bind to actin but the Ca^{2+}-affinity of troponin is changed only by the attachment of these crossbridges to actin.

Is the change in Ca^{2+}-sensitivity related to an alteration of myofilament spacing?

Although there is some evidence that the Ca^{2+}-affinity of troponin varies with SL (see above), it is not known how the changes in SL bring about the changes in the Ca^{2+}-affinity of troponin. One possible mechanism derives from changes in the spacing between thick and thin filaments as the SL is altered. Matsubara & Elliott[21] first showed that, in skinned skeletal muscles, as the SL is increased the interfilament spacing decreases. Similar changes in

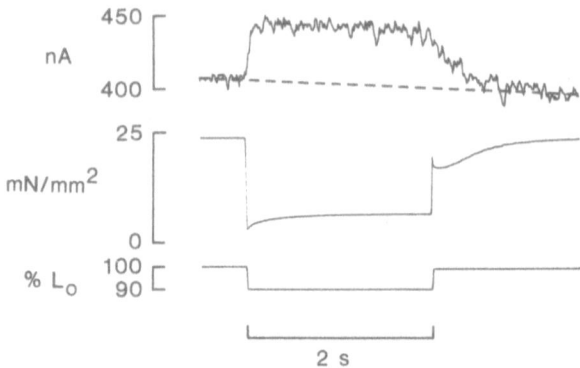

Fig. 4. Chart records of light emission from aequorin (top), force (middle), and muscle length (bottom) in a detergent)skinned trabecula from ferret ventricle. Prior to this, the muscle had been loaded with aequorin for 10 min and had then been activated to about 80% of maximum force with a solution of 15 μM Ca^{2+}. Averaged record from 16 length)changes. (From Allen & Kentish,[18] with permission.)

the lattice probably occur in skinned cardiac fibers. In skinned skeletal fibers, the effects of a decrease in filament spacing at constant SL have been investigated by Godt & Maughan,[22] who produced osmotic shrinkage of the myofilament lattice by adding to the bathing solutions long-chain polymers such as Dextran, which are excluded from the lattice. Godt & Maughan found that shrinkage of the lattice in 5% Dextran produced a large increase in myofibrillar Ca^{2+}-sensitivity (although a further increase of Dextran concentration from 5% to 10% decreased the Ca^{2+}-sensitivity so that it was the same as in the absence of Dextran; see also Fabiato & Fabiato[23]). Thus it seemed possible that the increased Ca^{2+}-sensitivity at longer SLs in skeletal and cardiac muscle is a result of a small decrease in filament spacing, similar to that produced by 5% Dextran.

To test this possibility in cardiac muscle, the Ca^{2+}-sensitivity of skinned cardiac trabeculae was measured during compression of the myofibrils with 5% and 10% Dextran at constant muscle length (Fig. 5). As in skinned skeletal fibers,[22] 5% Dextran increased maximum force slightly whereas 10% Dextran produced a small inhibition of force. However, in contrast to the skinned muscle studies, neither 5% nor 10% Dextran caused any change in the Ca^{2+}-sensitivity: the $[Ca^{2+}]$ for half-maximal activation was (in μM) 4.2 ± 0.5, 4.1 ± 0.7 and 4.3 ± 0.5 in the presence of 0%, 5% and 10% Dextran, respectively (mean ± s.e.m. of 3 muscles). Although lattice dimensions were not measured directly, it was clear that these concentrations of Dextran were causing considerable myofibrillar compression because they decreased muscle diameter by 12% (5% Dextran) and by 20% (10% Dextran), and the force responses to length changes were much slower, indicating an increased resistance to sarcomere shortening (results not shown).

From these results it would seem that in skinned cardiac muscle there is no

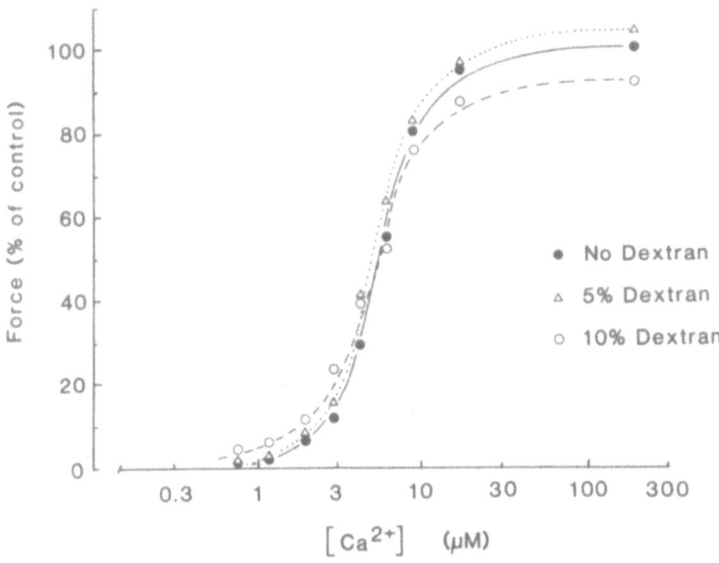

Fig. 5. Effect of myofibril compression with Dextran T-500 on the Ca^{2+}-sensitivity of a skinned trabecula from rat ventricle. Dextran was added to concentrations shown (g/100 ml). Solution composition similar to that for Fig. 1B. Forces are expressed relative to the maximum force in the absence of Dextran. Similar results were found in two other muscles. (Kentish, unpublished observations.)

effect of myofibrillar compression on Ca^{2+}-sensitivity. This makes it unlikely that the SL-dependence of Ca^{2+}-sensitivity in cardiac muscle depends upon the changes in myofilament lattice spacing with SL.

Thus at the moment it is not clear how SL influences the Ca^{2+}-affinity of troponin, although crossbridge attachment may be an intermediate step. As SL is reduced from 2.3 μm to 1.6 μm, there may be a small decrease (5%–15%) in the number of cycling crossbridges[10] (Fig. 2B), possibly due to steric hindrance from the double overlap of thin filaments, as first suggested by Gordon, Huxley & Julian.[1] This reduction of crossbridge number could then decrease the Ca^{2+}-affinity of troponin and the Ca^{2+}-sensitivity of the myofibrils. However, it seems unlikely that such a small decrease in the number of attached crossbridges could produce such large changes in Ca^{2+}-sensitivity as observed in the present experiments (Fig. 3). Thus the mechanism underlying the SL-dependence of myofibrillar Ca^{2+}-sensitivity remains to be established, although evidence is presented here that changes in the Ca^{2+}-affinity of troponin may be involved.

Conclusions

It is possible to identify several factors that may contribute to the steepness of the SL–force relationship in intact cardiac muscle (see Fig. 6): (A) There may be a small contribution from a decrease in the maximum force generated by the myofibrils at shorter sarcomere lengths, possibly because of a small reduction in the number of active crossbridges (Fig. 2b), or because other intracellular structures linked to the myofibrils generate an opposing force.[24] (B) Opposing forces, due to deformation of cells and extracellular structures such as collagen, could produce a large reduction of maximum force production in multicellular preparations such as trabeculae and probably also in the intact ventricular wall. The combination of factors (A) and (B) can result in a fairly steep SL–force relationship in trabeculae even at maximally-activating $[Ca^{2+}]$ (Fig. 1b). (C) At submaximal $[Ca^{2+}]$, the decrease in Ca^{2+}-sensitivity at shorter sarcomere lengths causes the curves to be steeper than at maximal $[Ca^{2+}]$; another consequence of this factor is that the curvature of

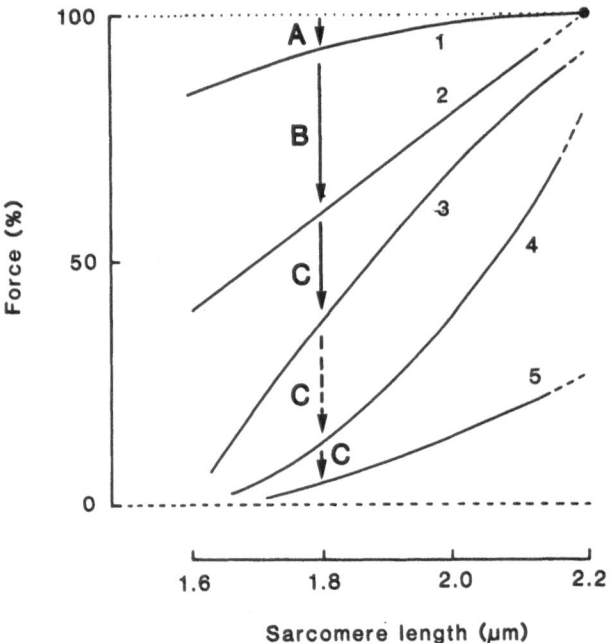

Fig. 6. Diagrammatic representation of SL–force relationships in different preparations from cardiac muscle: (1) maximally-activated skinned single cells;[24] (2) maximally)activated skinned cardiac trabeculae (from Fig. 1B); (3),(4),(5) submaximally-activated cardiac trabeculae (from Fig. 1B) or intact cardiac trabeculae (from Fig. 1A) at different $[Ca^{2+}]$. All curves normalized to the maximum Ca^{2+}-regulated force measured at SL = 2.2 μm in the same type of preparation. It is suggested that factors responsible for the decrease in force at shorter SL are:

(A) Intramyofibrillar, due to fewer active crossbridges, and intracellular, due to restoring forces arising in cellular structures such as the cytoskeleton or the sarcoplasmic reticulum (Fabiato & Fabiato, 1976).

(B) Extracellular, due to opposing forces produced by connective tissue and intercellular connections.

(C) Submaximal Ca^{2+}-activation in combination with the SL-dependence of myofibrillar Ca^{2+}-sensitivity.

the SL–force relationship depends upon the $[Ca^{2+}]$ (Figs. 1B and 6) i.e. upon the degree of potentiation in the muscle.

These factors in combination result in SL–force curves for the skinned muscles at submaximal $[Ca^{2+}]$ that are steep enough to explain the curves in the intact muscles (Fig. 1B). Thus the SL–force curves for the intact muscles may be largely due to the properties of the myofibrils and connective tissue in the preparation. However, it cannot be ruled out that other factors play an additional part. For example, there may be a contribution from the mechanical constraints imposed by the cell membranes of the intact cells, or there may be a SL-dependence of the Ca^{2+} release from the sarcoplasmic reticulum. Nevertheless, it would appear that these other factors may be of relatively limited significance and that a large part of the SL–force relationship of intact muscle can be explained by the properties of the myofibrils and connective tissue.

It should be borne in mind that this conclusion applies to the SL-force relationship in the intact muscle when the slow time-dependent changes of twitch force have not been allowed to occur (e.g. in the experiments of Fig. 1A); these slow changes, which occur in a time-scale of minutes after a change in muscle length and which tend to make the SL–force relationship even steeper,[7] are due to an additional mechanism that involves a progressive alteration in the magnitude of the Ca^{2+} transient.[8]

References

1. Gordon AM, Huxley AF and Julian FJ (1966). The variation in isometric tension with sarcomere length in vertebrate muscle fibers. J Physiol 184: 170–192.
2. Kentish JC, ter Keurs HEDJ, Ricciardi L, Bucx JJJ and Noble MIM (1986). Comparison between the sarcomere length–force relations of intact and skinned trabeculae from rat right ventricle. Circ Res 58: 755–768.
3. Fabiato A (1981). Myoplasmic free calcium concentration reached during the twitch of an intact isolated cardiac cell and during calcium)induced release of calcium from the sarcoplasmic reticulum of a skinned cardiac cell from the adult rat or rabbit ventricle. J Gen Physiol 78: 457–497.
4. ter Keurs HEDJ, Rijnsburger WH, van Heuningen R and Nagelsmit MJ (1980). Tension development and sarcomere length in rat cardiac trabeculae. Evidence of length-dependent activation. Circ Res 46: 703-714.
5. Krueger JW and Pollack GH (1975). Myocardial sarcomere dynamics during isometric contraction. J Physiol 251: 627–643.
6. Parmley WW and Chuck L (1973). Length-dependent changes in myocardial contractile state. Am J Physiol 224: 1195–1199.
7. Jewell BR (1977). A reexamination pf the the influence of muscle length on myocardial performance. Circ Res 40: 221–230.
8. Allen DG and Kurihara S (1982). The effects of muscle length on intracellular calcium transients in mammalian cardiac muscle. J Physiol 327: 79–94.
9. Kentish JC (1984). The inhibitory effects of monovalent ions on force development in detergent)skinned ventricular muscle from guinea)pig. J Physiol 352: 353–374.

10. Fabiato A and Fabiato F (1975). Dependence of the contractile activation of skinned cardiac cells on the sarcomere length. Nature 256: 54–56.
11. Winegrad S and Robinson TJ (1978). Force generation among cells in the relaxed heart. Eur J Cardiol 7 (Suppl.): 63–70.
12. Daniels M, Noble MIM, ter Keurs HEDJ and Wohlfart B (1984). Velocity of sarcomere shortening in rat cardiac muscle: relationship to force, sarcomere length, calcium and time. J Physiol 355: 367–381.
13. Kentish JC (1986). The effects of inorganic phosphate and creatine phosphate on force production in skinned muscles from rat ventricle. J Physiol 370: 585–604.
14. Kawai M and Brandt PW (1976). Two rigor states in skinned crayfish single muscle fibers. J Gen Physiol 68: 267–280.
15. Fabiato A (1980). Sarcomere length dependence of calcium release from the sarcoplasmic reticulum of skinned cardiac cells demonstrated by differential microspectrophotometry with Arsenazo III (abstr.) J Gen Physiol 76: 15a.
16. Hibberd MG and Jewell BR (1982). Calcium) and length-dependent force production in rat ventricular muscle. J Physiol 329: 527–540 (1982).
17. Allen DG and Kentish JC (1985a). The cellular basis of the length) tension relationship in cardiac muscle. J Mol Cell Cardiol 17: 821–840.
18. Allen DG and Kentish JC (1985b). The effects of length changes on myoplasmic calcium concentration in skinned ferret ventricular muscle. J Physiol 366: 67P.
19. Steiger GJ (1977). Tension transients in extracted rabbit heart muscle preparations. J Mol Cell Cardiol 9: 671–685.
20. Bremel RD and Weber A (1972). Cooperation within actin filament in vertebrate skeletal muscle. Nature New Biology 238: 101.
21. Matsubara I and Elliott GF (1972). X-ray diffraction studies on skinned single fibers of frog skeletal muscle. J Mol Biol 72: 657–669.
22. Godt RE and Maughan DW (1981). Influence of osmotic compressionon calcium activation and tension in skinned muscle fibers of the rabbit. Pflugers Archiv 391: 334–337.
23. Fabiato A and Fabiato F (1978). Myofilament)generated tension oscillations during partial activation and activation dependence of the sarcomere length)tension relation in skinned cardiac cells. J Gen Physiol 72: 667–699.
24. Fabiato A and Fabiato F (1976). Dependence of calcium release, tension generation and restoring forces on sarcomere length in skinned cardiac cells. Eur J Cardiol 4(Suppl. 13): 13–27.

Appendix

We append a comment kindly communicated to us by Dr. A. Fabiato concerning the lack of evidence for a length dependence of calcium)induced release of calcium from the cardiac sarcoplasmic reticulum:

Kentish et al.[1] have demonstrated that the length dependence of the sensitivity of the myofilaments to calcium could account for the ascending limb of the length tension diagram in the intact cardiac muscle. Our previous work had suggested that in addition to the length dependence of the sensitivity of the myofilaments to calcium, which we have observed,[2,3,4] there could be also a length dependence of calcium-induced release of calcium from the sarcoplasmic reticulum.[3,4,5,6] However, Allen and Kurihara[7] have demonstrated no immediate effect of a length change on the calcium transient detected with aequorin in intact cardiac muscle and Allen and Kentish[8] have found that the first calcium transient following an increase of length was in fact decreased in amplitude, which would be consistent with an increase of calcium binding to the myofilaments. This "personal communication" explains why there is in fact no evidence for a length dependence of calcium-induced release of calcium from the sarcoplasmic reticulum of a skinned cardiac cell (a fragment of a single cardiac cell from which the sarcolemma has been removed by microdissection).

Our first evidence for a length dependence of calcium-induced release of calcium from the cardiac sarcoplasmic reticulum of a skinned cardiac cell from the rat ventricle was based on experiments using tension recording to measure the increase of myoplasmic free calcium concentration resulting from the calcium release from the sarcoplasmic reticulum.[5] We were aware at this time of the data of Endo[9,10] demonstrating a length dependence of the sensitivity of the myofilaments to calcium in skinned fibers from skeletal muscle. However, as indicated in a subsequent article,[2] we thought that we had demonstrated that this phenomenon did not exist in skinned cardiac cells from the rat ventricle. We subsequently found out that our failure to confirm Endo's[9,10] results was related to an artifact caused by the unloading of the stiff parallel elastic element of skinned cardiac cells from the rat ventricle because of the imperfect isometry during contraction.[2] This resulted in a decrease of tension during the contraction which masked the length dependence of the sensitivity of the myofilaments to calcium. When we used skinned cardiac cells from other animal species, which were less stiff, it was possible to demonstrate a length dependence of the sensitivity of the myofilaments to calcium during partial calcium activation both at sarcomere length greater than 2.2 μm^2 and at sarcomere length shorter than 2.2 μm.[3,4,6] A more complete study of the length dependence of the calcium release in the ascending phase of the length-tension diagram has been reported by Hibberd and Jewell.[11,12]

Inasmuch as there is a length dependence of the sensitivity of the myofilaments to calcium, our original demonstration of a length dependence of calcium-induced release of calcium from the sarcoplasmic reticulum[5] is no longer valid: the sensor for detecting calcium release (i.e., the tension developed by the myofilaments) is itself sensitive to length. Accordingly, the calcium release had to be detected directly rather than through tension recording. This has been attempted in experiments reported in two abstracts.[3,4] The major purpose of this "personal communication" is to explain why these abstracts will not be submitted as full length articles.

Light absorption measurements with Arsenazo III provided some evidence for an increase of the amplitude of calcium-induced release of calcium when sarcomere length was increased[3] but the data were open to a number of possible artifacts because the light path was extremely small since the preparation was very thin. In addition, to avoid contraction artifacts the myosin of the skinned cell had to be extracted by exposure of the preparation to a high ionic strength. Finally, the data were exposed to the same artifacts caused by the method of activation of the preparation as will be explained for the results obtained with aequorin to detect calcium release.

Preliminary experiments done with aequorin in skinned cardiac cells from the canine ventricle[5] seemed to support the hypothesis of a length dependence of calcium-induced release of calcium in this preparation inasmuch as they showed an increase of the amplitude of the first calcium transient following an increase of sarcomere length. The method of activation of the skinned canine ventricular cells was by the system of rapid microinjections and microaspirations as described in Fabiato.[6] This method had been tested only for skinned cells from the canine Purkinje tissue in which there are fewer structures maintaining the myofibrils together than in the skinned canine working ventricular tissue. I thought, however, that the controls done in skinned canine Purkinje cells were likely to apply to other cardiac tissues, but intended to verify it before submitting this abstract for publication as a full length paper. Two types of findings were obtained during these control experiments which explain why I will not submit this abstract for publication. First, I found that the technique of rapid solution changes could not be safely applied to the working ventricular myocardium of the dog or the rat because the skinned cells from this tissue contains remaining pieces of transverse tubules and perhaps other structures preventing the broad separation of the myofibrils, which is essential for the rapid change of the solution bathing the outer surface of the sarcoplasmic reticulum. Secondly, no length dependence of calcium-induced release of calcium was observed in skinned canine Purkinje cells for which the technique of rapid solution changes was appropriate and had been thoroughly tested. In 35 experiments in skinned canine cardiac Purkinje cells I found no effect of the increase of sarcomere length from 1.7 μm to 2.2 μm on the first calcium-triggered calcium transient following this increase of sarcomere length in 23 cases, and a small decrease of this calcium transient in 12 cases.

The mechanism of the length dependence of the transient calcium signal observed in the skinned canine working ventricular cells with aequorin[4,6] and in the rat ventricular cells after myosin extraction with Arsenazo III[3] is not yet completely clear. An interesting possibility, suggested by Lakatta,[13] is that the increase of length which also decreases the thickness of the preparation may facilitate the diffusion of externally applied solutions. Since calcium-induced release of calcium is facilitated by a more rapid solution change at the outer surface of the sarcoplasmic reticulum,[6] the increase of length may cause an artifactual increase of the amplitude of the calcium-induced release of calcium.

Thus, at the present time there is no longer any argument in support of a length dependence of calcium-induced release of calcium from the cardiac sarcoplasmic reticulum. Consequently the explanation of the ascending limb of the length tension diagram by a length dependence of the sensitivity of the myofilaments to calcium proposed by Kentish et al.,[1] is entirely valid and no longer challenged by my data. I would have preferred to have more time to ascertain this negative conclusion before reporting it. Yet, it was urgent to communicate it, even in an inconclusive form to investigators working on the mechanism of Starling's Law of the Heart. Accordingly, the book edited by Drs. H.E.D.J. ter Keurs and M.I.M Noble seemed a most appropriate place for this "personal communication".

References

1. Kentish JC, ter Keurs HEDJ, Ricciardi L, Buckx JJJ and Noble MIM (1986). Comparison between the sarcomere length-force relations of intact and skinned trabeculae from rat light ventricle. Circ Res 58: 755–768.
2. Fabiato A and Fabiato F (1978). Myofilament)generated tension oscillations during partial calcium activation and activation dependence of the sarcomere length)tension relation of skinned cardiac cells. J Gen Physiol 72: 667–699.
3. Fabiato A (1980). Sarcomere length dependence of calcium release from the sarcoplasmic reticulum of skinned cardiac cells demonstrated by differential microspectrophotometry with Arsenazo III (Abstract). J Gen Physiol 76: 15a.
4. Fabiato A (1985a). Use of aequorin to demonstrate dependence of calcium)induced release of calcium from the sarcoplasmic reticulum of a skinned cardiac cell on active sarcomere length (Abstract). Biophys J 47: 378a.
5. Fabiato A and Fabiato F (1975). Dependence of the contractile activation of skinned cardiac cells on the sarcomere length. Nature, Lond. 256: 54–56.
6. Fabiato A (1985b). Rapid ionic modifications during the aequorin) detected calcium transient in a skinned canine cardiac Purkinje cell. J Gen Physiol 85: 189–246.
7. Allen DG and Kurihara S (1982). The effects of muscle length on intracellular calcium transients in mammalian cardiac muscle. J Physiol, Lond. 327: 79–94.
8. Allen DG and Kentish JC (1985). The effects of length changes on the myoplasmic calcium concentration in skinned ferret ventricular muscle. J Physiol, Lond. 366: 67p.
9. Endo M (1972). Stretch)induced increase in activation of skinned muscle fibres by calcium. Nature (New Biol) 327: 211–213.
10. Endo M (1973). Length dependence of activation of skinned muscle fibers by calcium. Cold Spring Harbor Symp Quant Biol 37: 505–510.
11. Hibberd MG and Jewell BR (1979). Length-dependence of the sensitivity of the contractile system to calcium in rat ventricular muscle (Abstract). J Physiol 290: 30–31p.
12. Hibberd MG and Jewell BR (1982). Calcium) and length-dependent force production in rat ventricular muscle. J Physiol, Lond. 329: 527–540.
13. Lakatta EG (1986). Length modulation of muscle performance: Frank) Starling law of the heart. In Heart and Cardiovascular System, Fozzard HA, Haber E, Jennings RB, Katz AM and Morgan HE (eds), pp 819–844, New York, Raven Press.

2. The Mechanism of the Length–Tension Relation in Cardiac Muscle of Rana Catesbeiana

TATSUO IWAZUMI

Department of Medical Physiology, University of Calgary, Alberta, Canada

Abstract

A recently developed instrument permits tension measurement and length control at such high resolution and frequency bandwidth that it is now possible to obtain static and dynamic mechanical properties of single myofibrils consisting of only 20 to 30 sarcomeres. Isometric tension vs. sarcomere length curves of bull-frog single or double myofibrils were constructed with intracellular solutions having pCa values of 9.0, 6.0, 5.5 and 5.0 at several sarcomere lengths from 2.2 μm to 3.6 μm. Every sarcomere of the myofibril preparation was observable and if a noticeable abnormality in sarcomere length uniformity and A-band misregistration developed, the data were rejected. Good quality single myofibrils produced up to 50 μg active tension which corresponds to about 5 Kg/cm^2 (or 50 N/cm^2). All active isometric tension vs. sarcomere length curves had positive slopes, i.e. active tension increased with sarcomere length up to 3.6 μm except when pCa was 5.0 in which case the tension measurements at greater sarcomere lengths than 3.0 μm were not possible without compromising the sarcomere uniformity and A-band registration. It was concluded that sarcomeres (both cardiac and skeletal) have an intrinsic property that the active tension increases with sarcomere length within the range of myofilament overlap so long as sarcomeres are activated by submaximal levels of Ca^{2+} concentration, and that excessive activation leads to misregistration of the A-band which appears to occur due to functional failure of myosin molecules.

Introduction

The "Frank-Starling relation" describes the output-volume relation of the heart which is represented by curves with positive slopes. When it is translated into the behavior of the sarcomeres in myocardial cells, their tension-length

H.E.D.J. ter Keurs and M.I.M. Noble (eds), Starling's Law of the Heart Revisited. ISBN 978-94-010-7084-3

relation are also described by curves with positive slopes. It is well known in mechanics that positive slopes in force-length (or pressure-volume) relations assure dynamic stability of the system while negative slopes lead to instability. This fact may not seem surprising since the rest length of mammalian cardiac sarcomeres in situ is about 1.9 μm, and the working sarcomere lengths under non-pathological conditions assume a range from 1.6 to 2.3 μm,[5] ie, myofilaments are mostly in double overlap configuration; therefore, the tension-length relation has positive slopes. On the other hand, skeletal sarcomeres, which have very similar ultrastructures to cardiac sarcomeres, function in simple overlap configuration. In *intact* single skeletal fibers, it is well known that the *tetanic tension* vs. sarcomere length relation can be described by a curve with a negative slope which more or less conforms to the proportionality with the overlap length. However, when the *Ca-activated tension* vs. sarcomere length relations were investigated in skinned fibers, it became apparent that there was no simple relationship between the active tension and the overlap length; a family of curves with different slopes were drawn, one for each Ca^{2+} concentration. When activated by submaximal Ca^{2+} intact concentrations (<5 μM), which are relevant to twitch activations in intact muscle cells, the slopes were positive for the lower range of sarcomere lengths, then turned negative beyond about 3 μm.[1] Now, the question is whether we can accept such data as true and artifact free.

Tension measurement per se is highly reliable; tension transducers can be calibrated accurately, and their frequency responses are not a factor in this case. But the measurement of sarcomere length can be very misleading. Sarcomere length is usually measured by optical microscopy or laser diffraction only at a spot or two along the length of the preparation. If the millions of sarcomeres in the preparation are highly uniform in their lengths and tension producing capacities, then such spot measurement is justified and acceptable. However, in reality, no perfect preparation exists. It then becomes necessary to state at least the distribution of sarcomere lengths along the entire length of the preparation both in rest and contraction. But, unfortunately this has seldom been done. Nonuniformity of sarcomere length becomes particularly severe when skinned fibers are activated by high $[Ca^{2+}]$ solutions at longer mean sarcomere lengths above 3 μm. For example, even skinned fibers selected most carefully for their exceptional sarcomere uniformity at rest (3.2 ± 0.1 μm) can develop a peak to peak variation of ± 0.25 μm during contraction at 6.3 μM Ca^{2+} concentrations.[2] In such skinned fibers the active tension vs. sarcomere length curves had positive slopes in the entire range, ie, the maximum tension was reached at 3.2 μm. If no particular care was taken, the peak to peak variation could easily reach $+0.5$ μm. In other words, the vast majority of skinned fibers can develop sarcomere non-uniformity to such an extent that some sarcomeres are stretched beyond overlap length

(3.65 μm). The consequence is substantially reduced tension since those stretched-out sarcomeres can support tension only by passive elasticity and other sarcomeres which are producing active tension are shortened and develop less tension owing to the positive slope of the length-tension curve. That this is what actually happens can be demonstrated by measuring the sarcomere lengths of the contracting fiber from end to end; the mean sarcomere length in contraction is much shorter than that at rest. The stretched-out sarcomeres escape detection by either microscopy or laser diffraction because all schemes of sarcomere length measurement rely upon the regularity of striation patterns; those out of the regularity are simply ignored.

There is another mechanism which reduces active tension of the sarcomere. It is structural distortion within the sarcomere. As shown in Fig. 1, when gross misregistrations of myofilaments take place, some of the thick and thin filaments are disengaged eventhough the sarcomere length is relatively short. The cause of the misregistration is of course a strong shear force between myofilaments but the mechanism of producing such a shear force is not well understood. The most likely explanation is localized failure of myosin heads, but detailed investigations are needed to explore this.

One might question the relevance of a positive slope in the tension-length relation at long sarcomere lengths since, after all, cardiac cells have strong passive elasticity which would prevent sarcomeres from being stretched beyond 2.3 μm. That this argument is incorrect can be seen in pathological cardiac sarcomeres some of which are stretched beyond filament overlap length while others are in super contracture, all mingled within a cell, i.e., individual sarcomeres are not constrained by a stiff elastic structure. The passive stiffness of amphibian cardiac myofibrils is similar to that of skeletal myofibrils as we shall see below. It seems nature's wisdom that the operating range of cardiac sarcomere length was chosen to be as far away as possible from the catastrophic event of thick and thin filament disengagement. In order to confirm that proposition, we must see that the cardiac sarcomere has tension-length curves with positive slopes extending all the way to the end limit of the overlap. As was the case for skinned skeletal fibers, large skinned cardiac cells are not satisfactory preparations for the intended experiment;

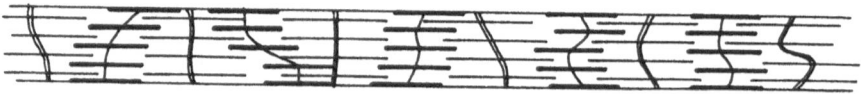

Fig. 1. Myofilament misregistrations and loss of overlap.When large shear forces develop between myofilaments the sarcomere structure becomes distorted and eventually develops disengagement of some thick and thin filaments. A likely cause of the shear force is local failures of myosin molecules.

they contain far too many sarcomeres to visually make sure of the sarcomere uniformity and good registration of the A-band. Therefore, we need to use cardiac myofibrils with only 20 to 30 sarcomeres so as to observe the behavior of every one of them.

Methods

Instrumentation

Two essential requirements for the measurement of the single myofibril mechanics are to measure forces in piconewtons and to control the myofibril length in nanometers, both on a time scale of microseconds. To satisfy these requirements special transducers were developed. The technical details may be found elsewhere[3] and only the working principle and summary of the system performance are described below.

Two very fine wires (12 μm diameter) are suspended in parallel, and a magnetic field is applied perpendicularly to the plane which includes both wires. The magnified image (50×) of each wire is projected onto a photo position detector which contains two parallel photodiodes with a very narrow gap. The wire position is determined by the normalized difference of two photo currents of the detector. The wires are insulated by polystyrene, and a single or double myofibril is mounted onto and perpendicular to the two wires using a very small amount of silicone adhesive (non-acid type). One of the wires serves as a force transducer and another as a length control actuator. The force is measured by the current that needs to be passed through the wire to counteract the myofibril tension so as to hold the wire position stationary. High speed small displacements (up to 6 μm) can be imposed on the other wire by a similar servo loop as force transducer except that an error between position command signal and the wire position signal is applied to the servo amplifier. The key performance figures of the system are as follows:

Length controller
Absolute resolution: 0.02 nm/Hz over 0–5 KHz, 2 nm rms over 50 KHz.
Step response: 10 μs.
Frequency response: 50 KHz with servo, 2 KHz without servo.

Force transducer
Absolute resolution: 0.5 ng/Hz (5 pN/Hz) over 0.5 KHz.
Frequency response: 50 KHz with servo, 2 KHz without servo.
Maximum force: 1 mg (10 μN).

Microdissections

Every step of the single myofibril experiment is critical, but the microdissection procedure is by far the most difficult and frustrating. Myofibrils were mechanically dissected by using super fine needles and four remotely controlled micromanipulators. Homogenization is a very simple method to produce myofibrils in large quantity, but they all suffer damage, even if they appear intact by optical microscopy, and show much less and slow development of tension compared with manually dissected good quality myofibrils. It is likely that the cause of the damage is excessive stretch of sarcomeres during homogenization since the manually dissected myofibrils also behaved similarly if their sarcomeres were stretched more than 50% of the slack length. When sarcomeres were excessively stretched the optical contrast of the A-band diminished even if they were promptly returned to the normal length, suggesting increased misregistration of the thick filaments.

Another scheme tried was to use enzymatically isolated myocytes which contain very few myofibrils, for example, bullfrog atrial cells. The extremities of these cells have only two myofibrils and are suitable for experiments. This preparation eliminates need of microdissection and is free from any possible damage by it, but instead the myofilaments were damaged nearly every time by the proteinase once the membrane was removed even after extensive washing of the cell.

Attachment of the myofibril to the transducers

The isolated myofibril is held down by two manipulation needles on the bottom of the chamber. The transducer with a very small bead of silicone adhesive is introduced into the chamber, then lowered onto the myofibril and gently rubbed against it until it is completely sunk into the adhesive. The entire mounting procedure must be completed within 30 seconds after the adhesive has formed a cone around the myofibril. Once hardened, the adhesive shows no deformation even at the maximum force at which the myofibril always breaks. Figure 2 shows a double myofibril mounted to the force and length transducers.

Solutions

The key parameters of the solutions were: pATP = 3 mM; pMg = 3 mM; pH = 7.10; u = 0.16; imidazole = 30 mM; CP = 12 mM; CPK = 1500 U/ml. The pCa values were 9.0, 6.0, 5.5, and 5.0. The flow control system had two

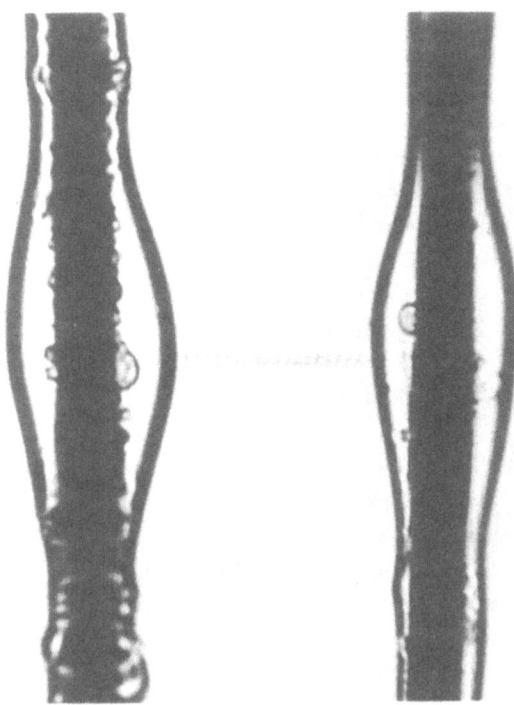

Fig. 2. Myofibril mounted between length (left) and force (right) transducers.This is a double myofibril from bullfrog atrium. Notice a thin tapered gap between the two single myofibrils. Two vertical rods are 12 μm diameter copper wires and the bulge is silicon adhesive.

reservoirs, one for the relaxing solution and another for the contracting solution, and these could be switched by remote control without creating a disturbance in the flow. A continuous flow was maintained at about 0.2 ml/min.

Results

The active tension vs. sarcomere length relations of a double myofibril from a bullfrog atrial cell are shown in Fig. 3. The top trace is a time course of the total myofibril tension starting with a rest at 2.2 μm (slack length), activation by pCa 5.5 at the same sarcomere length, relaxation, stretch to a new length 2.55 μm, activation by the same solution, relaxation, and so forth. The activation-relaxation cycles were always started at 2.2 μm, went up the sarcomere length values 2.55, 2.9, 3.25 and 3.6 μm, while stretches were made only during relaxed states, then came back down to 2.2 μm again. This protocol was repeated for each pCa value of 6.0, 5.5 and 5.0. The tension value at each sarcomere length was taken from the average of two measurements except at 3.6 µm to account for tension reduction due to myofibril deterioration.

The result is summarized in the lower part of Fig. 3. First, observe the passive tensions in the upper trace. At 3.25 µm it is about one quarter of the total tension. This proportion is comparable to or only a little higher than that observed in skinned skeletal fibers.[2] The slopes of active tension curves were all positive for pCa 6.0 and 5.5, but became nearly flat for 5.0 at sarcomere length above 2.9 µm. The myofibril could not withstand an activation by pCa 5.0 at 3.6 µm; it snapped off in the middle. In fact, this myofibril was only one among a large number of myofibrils tested that could maintain good sarcomere uniformity and registration during activation by pCa 5.0.

All other myofibrils tested developed sarcomere non-uniformity and A-band misregistration at 3.6 µm when activation by pCa 5.5. In other words, it was simply impossible to perform good experiments on myofibrils stretched to the near end of overlap and activated by high Ca^{2+} solutions *while maintaining sarcomere uniformity and A-band registration*. This may explain

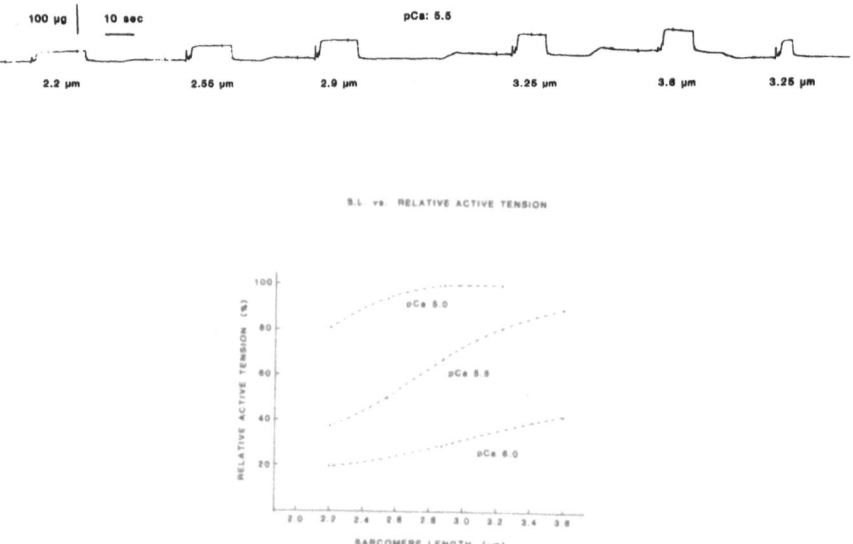

Fig. 3. A time course of myofibril tension undergoing series of contractions and active tension vs. length curves. The protocol is explained in the text. Note that the active tension rises in less than one second and relax in much less time. The tension rise time is a reliable indicator of the quality of the myofibril. If the myofibril has any problems which are not visually apparent the rise time often takes tens of seconds. The tension–length curves tend to be concave at low tension and become convex at high tension but their slopes are always positive so long as the sarcomere uniformity and registration are maintained.

why many investigators found diminishing tension values at long sarcomere lengths when skinned fibers were activated by high Ca^{2+} solutions; the sarcomeres of their preparations were in all probability not uniform nor well registered (sarcomere length distributions along the entire length of the preparation were not indicated in any of their results).

All good quality myofibrils in terms of sarcomere uniformity and A-band registration before the start of the experiments showed positive slopes in their tension-length curves without exception until they lost sarcomere uniformity on registration upon high tension development. Some myofibrils were stretched much beyond the overlap length and exposed to contracting solutions, but none developed active tension. Therefore, there must be a region, just beyond the end of overlap length, in which the active tension drops steeply. However, the tension measurements in this region always resulted in non-uniform contractures; it was not possible to perform repeatable experiments.

Another interesting finding was that the slack length of bullfrog myofibrils was always 2.2 μm, exactly the same slack length of skeletal myofibrils, although the "in situ" length before microdissection was about 1.9 μm. Therefore, the cardiac myofibril inside the cell is somewhat compressed in the longitudinal direction as well as in the transverse direction by the cytoskeleton and membrane.

The level of maximum active stress that myofibrils (both cardiac and skeletal) can produce were about 5 kg/cm² which is about twice as much as the stress normally found in skinned cardiac or skeletal muscles. Even if an ample allowance is made for their mitochondria and sarcoplasmic reticulum that occupy part of the cross-sectional area, the maximum active stress of the myofibril is substantially higher than those of large skinned preparations. This is another support for the importance of the sarcomere uniformity and myofilament registration to produce the maximal tension that the myofibril can produce.

Discussion

The cardiac myofibril experiments demonstrated that highly uniform and well registered sarcomeres indeed have tension-length curves with positive slopes in the entire range of sarcomere lengths where filament overlap is maintained so long as the activating solutions contain submaximal Ca^{2+} concentrations (<5 μM). The same was also true for skeletal myofibrils. However, even the best quality myofibrils could not withstand supramaximal Ca^{2+} concentrations (<10 μM); they always developed non-uniformity in the sarcomere lengths and misregistration in the A-band. It seems that very high active tension inflicts damage to the myosin molecules which results in many weak spots in the A-band. Indeed, flattening of tension-length curves at high tension may be an indication of myosin molecules reaching the limit of force generating capacity. Activations beyond the capacity would cause a damage to the myosin which then lose an active force, thus creating a large force imbalance with other myosin molecules resulting in high shear forces between the myofilaments.

Considering the level of active tension that intact cardiac muscle can produce in twitch contractions, the peak sarcoplasmic Ca^{2+} must be always submaximal. This is in agreement with the finding of other investigators.[4] It is then clear that the cardiac sarcomeres in normal conditions are operating on the tension-length curves whose slopes in the frog are always positive from 1.6 to 3.6 µm. Since the normal working range of sarcomere length in the mammalian heart is thought to be from 1.6 to 2.3 µm, one may postulate that, if no misregistration occurs, the cardiac sarcomere has a safety factor of almost 2 (1.3/0.7) before reaching the catastrophic failure due to myofilament disengagement. However, if the cell membrane is damaged thus permitting elevation of sarcoplasm Ca^{2+} concentration, then myofilament misregistration will increase significantly due to many myosin failures in the sarcomeres. This situation greatly reduces the safety factor; for example, if a misregistration of 0.65 µm occurs in any one of the many sarcomeres, the myofibril has no margin of safety at all even if their lengths are perfectly uniform. Now we can see why cardiac sarcomeres must operate at the lowest possible sarcomere lengths so as to reduce the chance of catastrophe as much as possible. Such an extra margin of safety may not be necessary for skeletal sarcomeres since a temporary failure is not life threatening.

If the slope of tension–length relation is so important for stable operation of muscle, one might question why most intact skeletal muscles operate in the negative slope region. The answer is fairly involved and not relevant to cardiac muscle; therefore, interested readers are referred to other work.[6,7,8,9] Another question as to a possible molecular mechanism by which myofilaments can produce greater active forces with less overlap is also answered in these papers.

In conclusion, the Frank-Starling's law in the heart is a manifestation of sound working principle of a mechanical system with a maximum margin of operating safety.

Acknowledgment

This research was supported in part by a grant-in-aid from the American Heart Association Texas Affiliate.

References

1. Stephenson DG and Wendt IR (1984). Length dependence of changes in sarcoplasmic calcium concentration and myofibrillar calcium sensitivity in striated muscle fibers. J Musc Res Cell Motility 5: 243–272.
2. Iwazumi T and Pollack GH (1981). The effect of sarcomere non-uniformity on the sarcomere length-tension relationship of skinned fibers. J Cell Physiol 106: 321–337.
3. Iwazumi T (1987). High-speed and ultra-sensitive instrumentation for myofibril mechanics measurements. Am J Physiol 252: C253–C262.
4. Fabiato A (1981). Myoplasmic free calcium concentration reached during the twitch of an intact isolated cardiac cell and during calcium-induced release of calcium from the sarcoplasmic reticulum of a skinned cardiac cell from the adult rat or rabbit ventricle. J Gen Physiol 78: 457–497.
5. Kentish JC, ter Keurs HEDJ, Ricciardi L, Bucx JJJ and Noble MIM (1986). Comparison between the sarcomere length-force relations of intact and skinned trabeculae from rat right ventricle. Circ Res 58: 755–768.
6. Iwazumi T (1970). A new field theory of muscle contraction. PhD Thesis, University of Pennsylvania. Univ Microfilms, Inc.
7. Iwazumi T (1978). Molecular mechanism of muscle contraction: another view. In: Cardiovascular system dynamics. Baan, Noordergraff and Raines (eds), MIT Press, 11–21.
8. Iwazumi T (1979a). A new field theory of muscle contraction. In: Crossbridge mechanism in muscle contraction. Pollack and Sugi, (eds), Univ. of Tokyo press: 611–632.
9. Iwazumi T (1979b). A theory of sarcomere dynamics. In: The cardiac cycle. MIM Noble, Blackwell: 54–89.

3. Intracellular Calcium Concentration Following Length Changes in Mammalian Cardiac Muscle

D.G. ALLEN, G.L. SMITH & C.G. NICHOLS

Department of Physiology, University of Maryland, Baltimore, Maryland, U.S.A.;
Department of Physiology, University College London, U.K.

Abstract

There is good evidence that activation of mammalian cardiac muscle is influenced by muscle length and that this length-dependent activation contributes to the shape of the length– tension relationship. Two mechanisms which could lead to such length-dependent activation are (i) changes in the amount of calcium supplied to the myofibrils and (ii) changes in the amount of calcium bound to the myofibrils for a given supply of calcium, e.g. by changes in the affinity of troponin for calcium. One way of studying length-dependent activation is to measure the intracellular calcium concentration in muscle during length changes. In this article we review the effects of changes in muscle length on intracellular calcium concentration in cardiac muscle and consider the mechanisms which may underlie them.

Introduction

One of the fundamental properties of all kinds of muscles is the way in which tension development depends on muscle length. In cardiac muscle this property has been recognised for at least a century and is enshrined in Starling's Law of the Heart (for a brief historical account, see Guz[1]). However, our understanding of the intracellular mechanisms which account for the length-dependence of tension remains incomplete (for recent reviews see Jewell,[2] ter Keurs,[3] Allen & Kentish[4]). Current theories suggest that both mechanical factors, such as myofilament overlap, and activation factors, such as the amount of calcium bound to troponin, are affected by muscle length and contribute to the length-dependence of tension.

H.E.D.J. ter Keurs and M.I.M. Noble (eds), Starling's Law of the Heart Revisited. ISBN 978-94-010-7084-3
© 1988, Kluwer Academic Publishers, Dordrecht

Mechanical factors

The work of Gordon, Huxley & Julian[5] identified changes in thick and thin filament overlap as the dominant mechanism on the descending limb (sarcomere length > 2.25 μm) of fully activated frog skeletal muscle. However on the ascending limb (sarcomere length < 2.0 μm) the interactions between thick and thin filaments are more complex and may involve restoring forces and the effects of interference between the overlapping ends of the thin filaments, as well as changes in overlap. At present no detailed model exists which relates tension and sarcomere length over the ascending limb in frog skeletal muscle.

The working range of mammalian cardiac muscle is restricted to sarcomere lengths between about 1.6 and 2.3 μm,[6] which constitutes the ascending limb of the length-tension relation. Studies in maximally activated skeletal single fibers[5] and maximally calcium-activated skinned cardiac muscle cells[7] have shown that, over this range of sarcomere lengths, the tension developed at the shortest length is about 80–90% of the maximum tension. However, in skinned cardiac trabeculae subject to maximal calcium-activation, reduction in sarcomere length from 2.1 to 1.6 μm reduced developed tension to 40% of the maximum.[8] The greater reduction in developed tension at short sarcomere lengths in trabeculae when compared to single cell was attributed by Kentish et al. to the presence of extracellular connective tissue in the trabeculae which could provide restoring forces at the short sarcomere lengths. Whatever the precise cause may be, the dependence of developed tension on sarcomere length in maximally calcium-activated preparations can be regarded as being due to mechanical factors. The important point is that in intact cardiac muscle, which is generally only partially activated, changes in sarcomere length over this range lead to even *larger* changes in developed tension. For instance, in the study of Kentish et al.,[8] reduction of sarcomere length from 2.1 μm to 1.6 μm in an intact trabecula led developed tension to fall to 0% of the maximum value. Thus the reduction in tension in intact, partially-activated muscles at short sarcomere lengths is greater than can be accounted for by mechanical factors; this finding was one of the earliest indications that changes in activation with muscle length might also contribute to the cardiac length-tension relation.

Activation factors

The term activation refers to all the processes which trigger contraction. These include the action potential, calcium entry across the surface membrane, calcium release from the sarcoplasmic reticulum (SR), the binding of calcium to troponin and the subsequent switching on of the actin sites leading to crossbridge cycling and tension development. The processes which subsequently lower the calcium level in the myoplasm leading to relaxation are also regarded as part of the activation cycle. These include reuptake of calcium into the sarcoplasmic reticulum and pumping of calcium back to the extracellular space. From the above summary it is clear that there are a large number of processes which could potentially be affected by muscle length and which would therefore lead to changes in activation.

Two independent mechanisms by which changes in length affect activation have so far been identified. (i) Changes in the affinity of troponin for calcium. Early evidence for this possibility came from studies by Endo[9] showing that the calcium-tension relation of skinned skeletal muscle was shifted to the left by increases in sarcomere length on the descending limb of the length–tension relation. This study was subsequently extended to the ascending limb of the cardiac length–tension relation.[10,8] Both studies showed that the apparent sensitivity of skinned cardiac muscle to calcium was increased by increases of sarcomere length within the normal working range. The simplest interpretation of this finding is that the affinity of troponin for calcium has been increased by stretch; as yet there is considerable circumstantial evidence for this interpretation but no direct proof. (ii) Changes in calcium release from the SR. This was first suggested by Parmley & Chuck[11] as an explanation for the slow changes in tension which they observed over 5–10 min following a length change. More recent evidence in favor of this idea came from the observation of increased calcium transients accompanying the slow increase in tension.[12] In addition, studies by Fabiato[13,14] using skinned cardiac cells have shown that calcium-induced calcium release from the SR is increased by stretch (but see his reservations in the Appendix to Chapter 1).

Measurements of $[Ca^{2+}]_i$ and tension following length changes

In the present article we will describe our own experiments in which free intracellular calcium concentration ($[Ca^{2+}]_i$) and tension have been measured in intact mammalian ventricular muscle during length changes. This experimental approach can be valuable in several ways. (i) Any change in $[Ca^{2+}]_i$ is a valuable indication that activation has been affected; however, it is not usually possible to identify unequivocally what change has occurred from this kind of experiment alone. For example, both a reduction in calcium release from the sarcoplasmic reticulum (SR) and an increase in the affinity of troponin for calcium will lead to a decrease in the size of the rise in free $[Ca^{2+}]_i$ during systole (the calcium transient). (ii) If, as seems inevitable, detailed investigation of the length-dependence of individual processes has to be done on isolated fragments of cells it is important to check that measurements in an intact preparation are compatible with the observations on the isolated organelles. For example, Fabiato[13,14] has data initially suggesting that calcium-induced calcium release from the SR is enhanced by stretch in skinned cell fragments; the relevance of this observation to intact preparations can potentially be assessed by observations of the calcium transients in intact muscle.

When muscle length is suddenly changed, developed tension changes in a complex way. We will consider the changes in tension and $[Ca^{2+}]_i$ on four separate timescales. For simplicity we will only describe the consequences of shortening muscle length. As a general rule lengthening produces the opposite effects to shortening; the main exception is the effects of sudden stretches during a contraction (see section (i) below). Though sarcomere length was neither measured nor controlled in the experiments we describe, more sophisticated mechanical experiments with sarcomere measurements and/or sarcomere clamping[15,16] have confirmed the main features of the tension changes we will describe.

$[Ca^{2+}]_i$ was measured using aequorin which was injected into many cells on the surface of the muscle. Aequorin is a protein which emits light when it binds calcium so that the resulting light signals are an indicator of $[Ca^{2+}]_i$. An important advantage of aequorin is that, provided light emission is collected with a detector which is large in comparison to the muscle size, the resulting signals are unaffected by movements of the muscle. For details of the aequorin technique, see Allen & Kurihara[12] and Cannell & Allen.[17] Muscle lengths are given as % L_{max}, where L_{max} is the length at which developed tension is maximal.

Interpretation of $[Ca^{2+}]_i$ and tension measurements

Aequorin measures the $[Ca^{2+}]_i$ which is the net result of all the processes which bring calcium into and which remove calcium from the intracellular space. Thus, as noted above, when $[Ca^{2+}]_i$ changes it is not necessarily easy to determine the mechanism(s) involved. Since there is already evidence for both changes in affinity of troponin for calcium and for changes in the release of calcium from the SR, it is worth considering how these might affect $[Ca^{2+}]_i$ and tension.

If troponin affinity increases this will lead to more calcium bound to troponin for a given $[Ca^{2+}]_i$. Assuming calcium release and entry to the myoplasm are unaffected, the net results will be a lower systolic $[Ca^{2+}]_i$ but more calcium bound to troponin and therefore more developed tension. If calcium release from the SR is increased this will lead to increases in systolic $[Ca^{2+}]_i$, in calcium bound to troponin and in developed tension.

These considerations show that when both $[Ca^{2+}]_i$ and tension are measured it is easy to distinguish between changes in troponin affinity and SR calcium release. The former leads to $[Ca^{2+}]_i$ and tension changing in opposite directions while the latter leads to parallel changes in $[Ca^{2+}]_i$ and tension.

(i) Rapid shortening during a contraction

If a large and rapid shortening is imposed on a muscle during a contraction, the immediate consequence is a rapid fall in developed tension to zero. The muscle then shortens at its maximum rate until the slack has been taken up and subsequently tension slowly redevelops (Fig. 1A, right hand panel). In mammalian cardiac muscle the level to which tension recovers is generally less than expected for the new time and length:[18] this phenomenon is known as shortening deactivation.

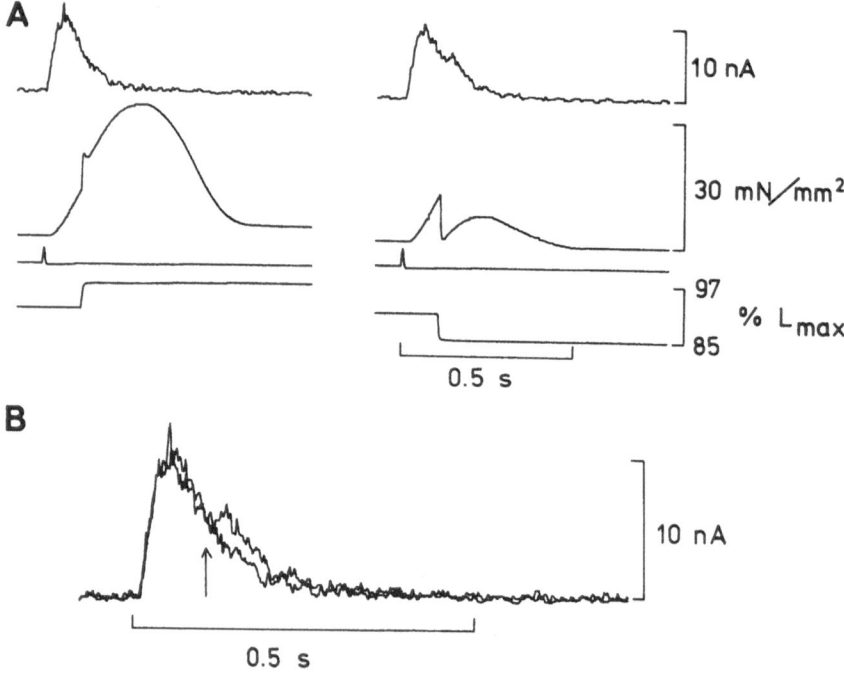

Fig. 1. Effect of a rapid stretch and rapid release on aequorin light ($[Ca^{2+}]_i$) and tension; cat papillary muscle, 30°C. Panel A shows from above down; light, tension, stimulus marker, muscle length. The left hand panel shows a stretch and the right hand panel a release. The length change was made 110 ms after the stimulus and the new length maintained for 1 s. Length was then returned to the control value for the remainder of the diastolic period. This sequence was repeated 64 times and averaged to obtain each figure. Panel B shows the two light signals from A superimposed; the arrow indicates the time of the length changes. Light signals from the control length (92% L_{max}) were not significantly different from the light signal of A but significantly different from B. Modified from Allen & Kurihara[12] with permission.

The intracellular calcium signal increases over the period in which tension is reduced and when rapid shortening is occurring. If the release occurs more slowly, the rise in $[Ca^{2+}]_i$ is smaller and slower.[19] Isotonic shortening also leads to an enhanced $[Ca^{2+}]_i$ during the period of shortening.[20,21,19] The increase in calcium is detectable about 10 ms after the shortening.[19] The subsequent time course is difficult to estimate, both because it is superimposed on a changing signal and because of the the non-linearity of aequorin signals: however, the increase in $[Ca^{2+}]_i$ appears to reach a peak after 20–30 ms and then declines. Similar signals have been observed in barnacle muscle.[22] Stretch leads to a fall in $[Ca^{2+}]_i$ but, as shown in Fig. 1A, the magnitude of the change is smaller than an equivalent shortening.

The rise in $[Ca^{2+}]_i$ which accompanies shortening (or reduced tension) could arise from many sources. Shortening could lead to increased SR calcium release or perhaps to enhanced calcium influx through the surface membrane. The latter possibility is consistent with the positive shift in the membrane potential which also occurs during shortening,[19,23] but the fact that changes in $[Ca^{2+}]_i$ seem to precede the changes in membrane potential[19] makes this mechanism unlikely. A further argument against the possibility that either increased calcium entry or increased SR calcium release are responsible for the rise of $[Ca^{2+}]_i$ is that the deactivation of tension suggests *less* calcium binding to troponin rather than more.

The combination of elevated $[Ca^{2+}]_i$ but depressed tension suggests that calcium has been displaced from troponin into the myoplasm, in other words that the affinity of troponin for calcium has fallen.[12,19,20] This explanation is consistent with skinned fiber studies which have shown that the apparent calcium sensitivity of a preparation is decreased at short muscle lengths.[8,10] Further support for this theory comes from recent work in which a rise of myoplasmic $[Ca^{2+}]_i$ has been observed in skinned fibers following a reduction in muscle length[24] (see also Chapter 1 by Kentish, ter Keurs & Allen, this volume). These fibers were skinned by prolonged exposure to the detergent Triton-X 100 and should be completely free of membrane, so that the rise of $[Ca^{2+}]_i$ cannot arise from any membrane source. An interesting feature of these experiments was that after shortening, the fall of tension and the rise in myoplasmic $[Ca^{2+}]$ were rapid. However, after stretching, developed tension took a substantial time (0.5–1 s) to redevelop and the myoplasmic $[Ca^{2+}]$ fell with a comparably slow time course. These observations may explain why stretch in an intact fiber apparently has less effect on $[Ca^{2+}]_i$ than shortening. If it is assumed that it is the changes in tension consequent on the length change which cause the changes in $[Ca^{2+}]_i$, then the slower response to stretch may mean that significant changes in $[Ca^2]_i$ do not have time to occur in the limited duration of a contraction.

The mechanism by which mechanical conditions affect the affinity of troponin for calcium remain unknown. On the basis of the experimental results available at present it appears that two mechanisms might be involved. Experiments in which a steady-state change in troponin affinity has been observed at different sarcomere lengths[8,10,24] show that sarcomere length has an effect on troponin affinity. Experiments in which active shortening occurs[12,19,20] have consistently shown that shortening rapidly between two lengths leads to a larger change in $[Ca^{2+}]_i$ than when the muscle contracts isometrically at the longest and shortest of the range of lengths involved. For the present we prefer to assume that only one mechanism is involved in both phenomena and that the fundamental factor is the number of crossbridges attached to the thin filament. There is good evidence to suppose that both at short sarcomere lengths and during active shortening[25] the number of attached crossbridges is reduced. A biochemical basis for a link between crossbridge attachment and the affinity of troponin for calcium is suggested by the work of Bremel & Weber.[26] They showed that the affinity of troponin for calcium in isolated thin filaments was increased when rigor crossbridges were attached to the thin filament. If this mechanism operates during the attachment of crossbridges during normal contraction, then any manoeuvre which reduces the number of crossbridges attached e.g. shortening will lower the troponin affinity. This will lead to a rise in $[Ca^{2+}]_i$ and a fall in developed tension. For a fuller discussion of this theory see Allen & Kentish.[4]

(ii) Changes in the first contraction following shortening

If a muscle length is reduced during diastole, the next contraction is smaller. When shortening is substantial, i.e. >10% muscle length, there is a detectable increase in the amplitude of the first calcium transient which accompanies the reduced tension (Fig. 2). There are also changes in the time course of both the calcium transient and the tension: the declining phase of the calcium transient is prolonged whereas the contraction is abbreviated.

The simultaneous decrease in tension and increase in $[Ca^{2+}]_i$ again suggest that the affinity of troponin for calcium has fallen at the shorter length. In a maximally calcium-activated muscle, tension falls to 40–50% of maximum when length is reduced from L_{max} to 80% L_{max}.[8] However, in the experiment illustrated in Fig. 2 tension has fallen to 5% of its maximum over this range of shortening so that the reduction in tension is much greater than can be accounted for by mechanical factors. It is this reduction in tension over and above that which can be accounted for by mechanical factors, coupled with an increase in systolic $[Ca^{2+}]_i$, which suggests that the troponin affinity for calcium must have fallen.

The abbreviation of the time course of tension and the prolongation of the

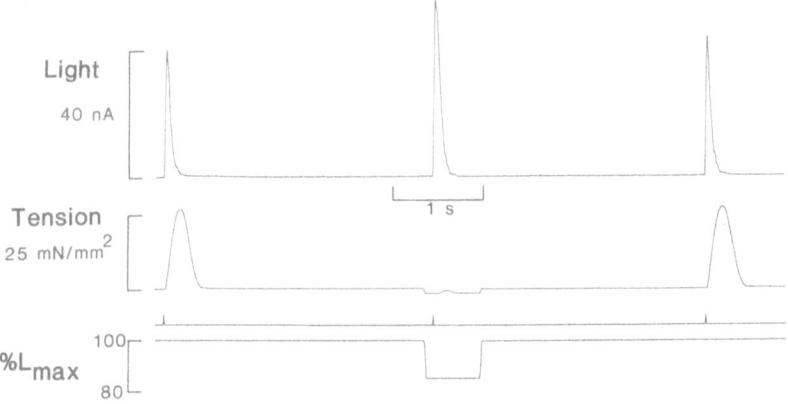

Fig. 2. The effect of a reduction in muscle length during the diastolic period on aequorin light ($[Ca^{2+}]_i$) and tension of the 1st contraction at the new length; ferret papillary muscle, 30°C. The muscle was held at the reduced length for one contraction and then returned to the control length for 6 contractions in order to minimize the development of slower consequences of length changes. This cycle was repeated 16 times and averaged to obtain the figure. Taken from Allen & Smith,[36] with permission.

time course of $[Ca^{2+}]_i$ are both also consistent with a reduction in the affinity of troponin for calcium. In this discussion we assume that the fall in troponin affinity arises from an increase in the rate for dissociation of calcium from troponin (off rate); the other possibility, that the association rate is decreased, seems less likely because this rate constant has the very high value of 10^8 s^{-1}. This indicates that it is diffusion controlled and unlikely to be influenced by physiological events. In the presence of a faster off rate, calcium will be removed from troponin more rapidly than otherwise and this will tend to abbreviate the time course of tension. The rate of decline of $[Ca^{2+}]_i$ tends to be slower because more calcium is released from troponin per unit time and the various calcium pumps therefore take longer to pump the calcium down to any given level.

While it is relatively easy to show that the above changes in tension and $[Ca^{2+}]_i$ are all consistent with a fall in the affinity of troponin for calcium at short lengths, the changes have not yet been analysed quantitatively. Our present hypothesis is that a combination of mechanical factors associated with the length change, together with the changes in troponin affinity, can explain all of the observations described above. However, this remains unproven. This is important in the context of the work of Fabiato[13,14] who has previously indicated that in skinned cardiac cells, calcium-induced calcium-release from the SR may increase immediately after a stretch. Our results in intact muscles do not support this possibility since we find the calcium transients *decreased* immediately after a stretch. Of course it is possible that both changes in release and affinity occur simultaneously; however, Fabiato now has doubts about his preliminary data (Appendix to

Chapter 1). If our hypothesis were sufficiently quantitative it would be possible to determine whether there were changes in calcium release in addition to the changes in troponin affinity.

(iii) Changes over 4–8 contractions

Developed tension in the first contraction after shortening is reduced but a small recovery is observed over the next 4–8 contractions (Fig. 3). This recovery is similar to the increase in magnitude of isotonic shortening which occurs over 4–8 contractions following a change from isometric to isotonic conditions. Housmans, Lee & Blinks[21] have shown that this increase in isotonic shortening is accompanied by an increase in the calcium transients. Figure 3 shows that the 4–8 beat recovery that follows shortening is also associated with a small increase (5–10%) in the calcium transients. Figure 3 also shows that the opposite sequence of changes occurs when the muscle is returned to the longer length. It is worth noting that muscles which are set to 80% L_{max} actually have a resting length longer than 80% because the length which the muscle takes up with no load (slack length) is typically 85–90% L_{max}. Thus muscles set to lengths shorter than the slack length will have a period of unloaded shortening before developing tension; in this respect changes in muscle length to below slack length resemble the change from isometric to isotonic conditions.

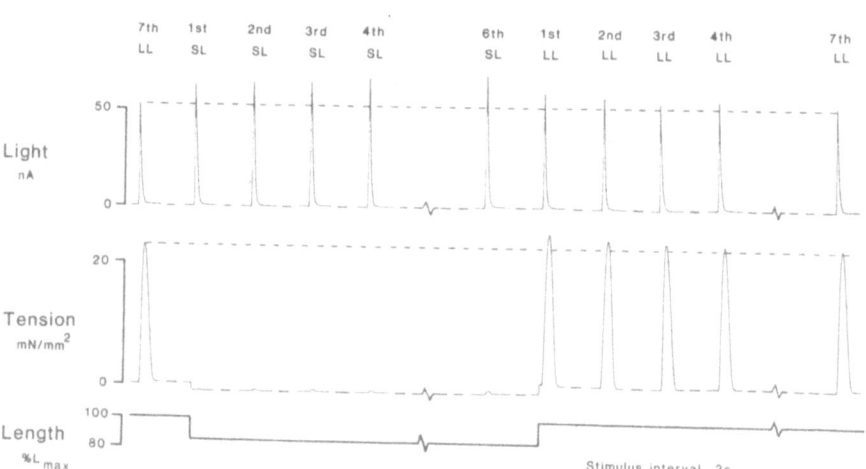

Fig. 3. Changes in aequorin light ($[Ca^{2+}]_i$) and tension on the first 4 contractions after a length change; ferret papillary muscle, 30°C, stimulus interval 3 s. The muscle was held at the long length (100% L_{max}) for 7 contractions and then shortened to 83% L_{max} for 6 contractions. The sequence was repeated 16 times and averaged to obtain the above figure. Part of each diastolic period and some of the contractions have been removed to reduce the size of the figure. Unpublished experiment of Allen & Smith.

During these 4–8 beat changes in tension the calcium transients and tension are changing in parallel and there are no changes in the time course of the Ca transient or the contraction. These observations suggest that changes in calcium release or entry to the myoplasm are the cause of the 4–8 beat effects. Changes in contractility with this time course are known to occur when the action potential is modified.[27] Thus in studies of the 4–8 beat effects associated with changing from isometric to isotonic conditions,[28,29] the changes in contractility were attributed to the changes in action potential duration which are known to accompany this mechanical change.[19,23] An important test of this theory would be to change the mechanical conditions of contraction under voltage clamp conditions, but this has not yet been achieved.

An alternative type of mechanism, in which the observed changes in action potential would be a secondary phenomenon rather than the direct cause of the changes in $[Ca^{2+}]_i$ and tension, arises from the changes in troponin affinity which occur when the length is changed. On the first contraction at the short length, the calcium transient is larger and more prolonged; consequently both calcium uptake by the SR and calcium extrusion from the cell will tend to be larger. This leads to two opposing effects; (i) increased SR calcium uptake tends to *potentiate* the subsequent SR calcium release and tension whereas (ii) increased extrusion from the cell will tend to deplete the cell of calcium and *reduce* subsequent calcium transients and tension. Preliminary modelling of this situation has shown that it is possible to make models in which either process dominates in the short term and it is not yet clear which model is physiologically more realistic.

(iv) Slow changes in $[Ca^{2+}]_i$ and tension after shortening

Following the small 4–8 beat recovery after shortening, developed tension then shows a substantial decline which takes 5–10 min to complete. These slow changes were first described by Parmley & Chuck[11] and subsequently shown to be accompanied by changes in the calcium transients as shown in Fig. 4. The reverse effects are seen after stretch. No changes in the time course of each individual calcium transient or the contractions occurred over this period.

The parallel changes in $[Ca^{2+}]_i$ and tension suggest that changes in calcium entry to the myoplasm, either from the SR or the surface membrane, are the cause of the slow changes in tension. Lakatta & Jewell[30] showed that the tension changes were attenuated by calcium blocking agents and proposed that the mechanism of these effects might involve changes in the calcium current. Recent experiments by Nichols,[31] however, suggest that it is the diastolic period which is important in triggering these effects. In the

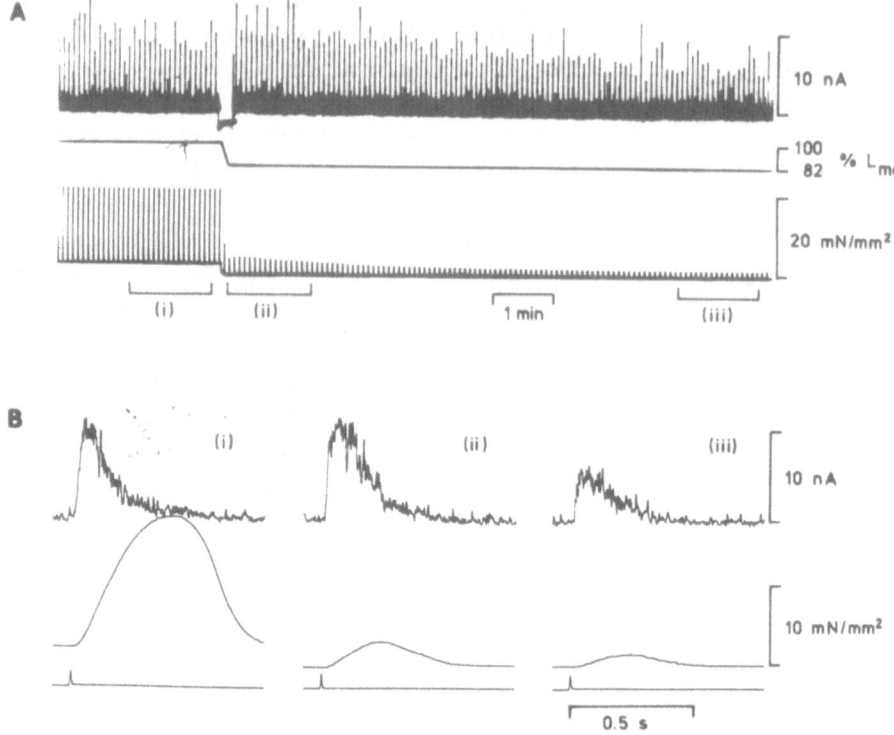

Fig. 4. Slow changes in aequorin light ($[Ca^{2+}]_i$) and tension following a reduction in muscle length; cat papillary muscle, 30°C. Panel A. Continuous record of light and tension before and after length change (the photomultiplier tube was turned off for about 20 s during the length change). Panel B. Averaged records of light and tension from 16 contractions during control period (i), immediately after length change (ii) and after 7 min at the short length (iii). Modified from Allen & Kurihara,[12] with permission.

experiments of Nichols the length of an isolated papillary muscle was controlled by a motor and changed rapidly before and after each systole. Muscle length could therefore be set to different values during systole and diastole. Nichols found that if systolic length was maintained at a control (long) length, but the muscle was held at a short length during the diastolic period, the developed tension showed a reduction of 20–40% over 5–10 minutes (this protocol is illustrated in Fig. 5). This reduction in developed tension is similar to the slow changes which would have been observed if the muscle had been held continuously at the short length. In the converse experiment, in which the muscle was held at a short length during systole but maintained at the long length during diastole, no such slow effects were observed. It therefore appears that the development of slow effects are a consequence of muscle length during diastole rather than systole. This conclusion was reinforced by experiments in which the muscle was held

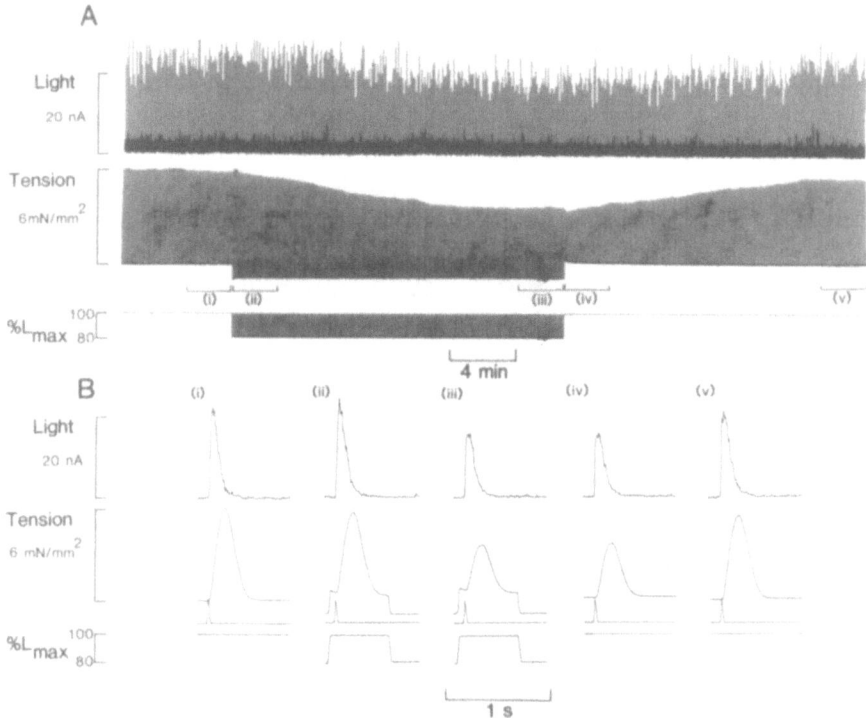

Fig. 5. Effect of diastolic shortening on aequorin light ($[Ca^{2+}]_i$) and tension; ferret papillary muscle, 30°C. Panel A. Continuous record of light, tension and muscle length. During the period of diastolic shortening the muscle was shortened about 100 ms after the contraction had relaxed and then held at this length until about 100 ms before the next contraction at which time it was restretched to the control length. Panel B shows records of light, tension, stimulus marker and muscle length obtained by averaging 32 contractions over the periods shown in Panel A. From Allen, Smith & Nichols,[32] with permission.

quiescent for 10 minutes and the subsequent recovery of tension observed.[31] If the muscle was shortened during the quiescent period, the developed tension during the recovery period was reduced compared with muscles whose length remained long during the quiescent period. The two recoveries approached each other over a period of 5–10 minutes. This experiment shows that simply holding the muscle at a short length, in the absence of any contraction, leads to a reduction of subsequent contractions over 5–10 minutes.

These results have now been extended by measuring the calcium transients during such manoeuvres.[32] The changes in calcium transients paralleled the changes in developed tension described above in all cases. A representative result is shown in Fig. 5 which illustrates the decline in developed tension and calcium transients when the muscle was shortened in the diastolic period but maintained at a long length during the systolic period.

The simplest interpretation of these results is that the resting $[Ca^{2+}]_i$ falls with a time course of 5–10 minutes when cardiac muscle is reduced in length. We have not been able to detect such a change in resting $[Ca^{2+}]_i$ reliably but this may simply reflect the difficulties of measuring resting $[Ca^{2+}]_i$ in cardiac muscles using aequorin. An effect of this kind has been observed by several groups in skeletal muscle, where muscle length can be changed over a much greater range.[33,34] On this hypothesis, the fall in resting $[Ca^{2+}]_i$ at short lengths leads to reduced SR calcium loading and hence to reduced calcium release, smaller calcium transients and reduced developed tension.

If such slow changes in resting $[Ca^{2+}]_i$ do occur in cardiac muscle there are many possible mechanisms which could be involved. The inward calcium leak into the cell might be increased by stretch; alternatively an increased inward sodium leak would raise $[Na^+]_i$ and this would lead to an elevated $[Ca^{2+}]_i$ by means of the Na/Ca exchanger in the surface membrane. There is evidence in embryonic cultured skeletal muscle cells for a stretch sensitive Na/K conductance which could conceivably underlie such an effect.[35]

Conclusions

The evidence that muscle length affects activation in cardiac muscle is overwhelming. At least two mechanisms are involved; (i) changes in calcium-affinity of the troponin and (ii) changes in SR calcium loading and release. Further understanding of the details of these processes will require studies on isolated components of the cardiac cells. This will enable the properties of these components to be studied without the complication of other aspects of cellular function. However, studies of the $[Ca^{2+}]_i$ and developed tension in intact cells will remain an important line of enquiry because such experiments indicate the overall response of the integrated cell whose function ultimately dictates the mechanical performance of the heart. In addition it is essential to check that properties observed and defined in isolated systems do indeed function in a similar fashion in the intact heart.

Acknowledgements

We thank Drs. Elliott, J.C. Kentish and J.A. Lee for valuable comments on the manuscript. This work was supported by grants from the Medical Research Council and the British Heart Foundation.

References

1. Guz A (1974). Chairman's introduction. The physiological basis of Starling's Law of the Heart. CIBA Foundation Symposium 24: 1–6. Elsevier, North-Holland.
2. Jewell BR (1977). A re-examination of the influence of muscle length on myocardial performance. Circ Res 40: 221–230.
3. ter Keurs HEDJ (1983). Calcium and contractility. In: Cardiac Metabolism, A.J. Drake-Holland & M.I.M. Noble (eds), pp 73–99. Chichester: John Wiley and Sons Ltd.
4. Allen DG and Kentish JC (1985b). The cellular basis of the length-tension relation in cardiac muscle. J Mol Cell Cardiol 17: 821–840.
5. Gordon AM, Huxley AF and Julian FJ (1966). The variation in isometric tension with sarcomere length in vertebrate muscle fibers. J Physiol 184: 170–192.
6. Page SG (1974). Measurements of structural parameters in cardiac muscle. In The Physiological Basis of Starling's Law of the Heart, pp.13–25. CIBA Foundation Symposium 24. Amsterdam: Elsevier (1968).
7. Fabiato A and Fabiato F (1975). Dependence of the contractile activation of skinned cardiac cells on the sarcomere length. Nature 256: 54–56.
8. Kentish JC, ter Keurs HEDJ, Ricciardi L, Bucx JJJ and Noble MIM (1986). Comparison between the sarcomere length-force relations of intact and skinned trabeculae from rat right ventricle. Circ Res 58: 755–768.
9. Endo M (1972). Stretch-induced increase in activation of skinned muscle fibers by calcium. Nature New Biology 237: 211–213.
10. Hibberd MG and Jewell BR (1982). Calcium- and length- dependent force production in rat ventricular muscle. J Physiol 329: 527–540.
11. Parmley WW and Chuck L (1973). Length-dependent changes in myocardial contractile state. Am J Physiol 224: 1195–1199.
12. Allen DG and Kurihara S (1982). The effects of muscle length on intracellular calcium transients in mammalian cardiac muscle. J Physiol 327: 79–94.
13. Fabiato A (1980). Sarcomere length dependence of calcium release from the sarcoplasmic reticulum of skinned cardiac cells demonstrated by differential microspectrophotometry with arsenazo III. J Gen Physiol 76: 15a.
14. Fabiato A (1985). Use of aequorin to demonstrate dependence of calcium-induced release of calcium from the sarcoplasmic reticulum of skinned cardiac cell on active sarcomere length. Biophysics Journal 47: 378a.
15. ter Keurs HEDJ, Rijnsburger WH, van Heuningen R and Nagelsmit MJ (1980). Tension development and sarcomere length in rat cardiac trabeculae. Evidence of length-dependent activation. Circ Res 46: 703–714.
16. Gordon AM and Pollack GH (1980). Effects of calcium on the sarcomere length-tension relation in rat cardiac muscle. Implications for the Frank-Starling mechanism. Circ Res 47: 610–619.
17. Cannell MB and Allen DG (1983). A photomultiplier tube assembly for the detection of low light levels. Pflugers Archiv 398: 165–168.
18. Brady AJ (1966). Onset of contractility in cardiac muscle. J Physiol 184: 560–580.
19. Lab MJ, Allen DG and Orchard CH (1984). The effects of shortening on myoplasmic calcium concentration and on the action potential in mammalian ventricular muscle. Circ Res 55: 825–829.
20. Housmans PK, Lee NK and Blinks JR (1983a). Active shortening retards the decline of the intracellular calcium transient in mammalian heart muscle. Science 221: 159–161.
21. Housmans PK, Lee NK and Blinks JR (1983b). History of loading in preceding contractions influences intracellular calcium transients in cat papillary muscle. Fed Procs 42: 573.
22. Ridgway EB and Gordon AM (1984). Muscle calcium transients; effects of post-stimulus length change in single fibers. J Gen Physiol 83: 75–104.
23. Kaufmann RL, Lab MJ, Hennekes R and Krause H (1971). Feedback interaction of mechanical and electrical events in the isolated mammalian ventricular myocardium. Pflugers Archiv 324: 100–123.

24. Allen DG and Kentish JC (1985a). The effects of length changes on the myoplasmic calcium concentration in skinned ferret ventricular muscle. J Physiol 366: 67P.
25. Julian FJ and Morgan DL (1981). Variation in muscle stiffness with tension during tension transients and constant velocity shortening in the frog. J Physiol 319: 193–203.
26. Bremel RD and Weber A (1972). Cooperation within actin filaments in vertebrate skeletal muscle. Nature, New Biology 238: 97–101.
27. Beeler GW and Reuter H (1970). The relation between membrane potential, membrane currents and activation of contraction in ventricular myocardial fibers. J Physiol 207: 211–229.
28. Parmley WM, Brutsaert DL and Sonnenblick EH (1969). Effects of altered loading conditions on ctractile events in isolated cat papillary muscle. Circ Res 24: 521–533.
29. Jewell BR and Rovell JM (1973). Influence of previous mechanical events on the contractility of isolated papillary muscle. J Physiol 235: 715–740.
30. Lakatta EG and Jewell BR (1977). Length-dependent activation: its effect on the length-tension relation in cat ventricular muscle. Circ Res 40: 251–257.
31. Nichols CG (1985). The influence of 'diastolic' length on the contractility of isolated cat papillary muscle. J Physiol 361: 269–279.
32. Allen DG, Nichols CG and Smith GL (1985). The effect of diastolic length on calcium transients in isolated ferret ventricular muscle. J Physiol 365: 57P.
33. Snowdowne KW and Lee NKM (1980). Subcontracture concentrations of potassium and stretch cause an increase in the activity of intracellular calcium in frog skeletal muscle. Fed Procs 39: 1733.
34. Lopez JR, Alamo L and Caputo C (1985). The increase in metabolic rate associated with stretching in skeletal muscle might be related to an increment in free $[Ca^{2+}]$. Biophysical Journal 47: 378a.
35. Guharay F and Sachs F (1984). Stretch-activated single ion channel currents in tissue-cultured embryonic chick skeletal muscle. J Physiol 352: 685–701.
36. Allen DG and Smith GL (1985). The first calcium transient following shortening in isolated ferret ventricular muscle. J Physiol 366: 83P.

4. Some Dynamic Effects of Length and Isotonic Motion on Cardiac Sarcomere Shortening

JOHN W. KRUEGER[1] & TAKAO OKADA[2]

[1]*Department of Physiology, Juntendo University Medical School, Tokyo, Japan*; [2]*The Albert Einstein College of Medicine, Bronx, New York, U.S.A.*

Abstract

The end point of isotonic shortening in isolated heart muscle is independent of initial sarcomere length *unless* the latter is longer than 2.0 µm at the onset of isotonic motion. An increase in force or a decrease in activation lengthens the sarcomere at peak shortening, but only so in direct proportion to the increment in sarcomere length above 2.0 µms at this time. Thus, a relatively simple relationship characterizes the complex interaction between length, force, and time to modify isotonic shortening in heart muscle. The instantaneous influence of length on the progressive slowing of shortening suggests that the effect of isotonic motion is equivalent to an increase in the internal load on the shortening sarcomere. An inactive region at the ends of the sarcomere, established by the time of the onset of isotonic motion, can explain how activation, nature of loading, and length might interact dynamically to influence variably the contractile performance of the heart. It has a further consequence for an equilibrium between activation and secondary adjustments in end diastolic volume.

Introduction

The end points of cardiac muscle shortening are primarily attributed to the static determined properties of the myofibrils. Thus, initial length does not affect the end points of cardiac sarcomere shortening which occurs early in contraction. However, the nonsteady aspect of cardiac muscle contraction implies that initial length will influence final length when shortening is a) delayed or b) slowed by load and/or intrinsic mechanisms.[1]

A major uncertainty in this situation is the influence of motion. For example, active shortening is thought to depress twitch contractions in striated muscle. This process is commonly known as "shortening deactivation". To rule out time as a factor, the depressive effect of active shortening

H.E.D.J. ter Keurs and M.I.M. Noble (eds), Starling's Law of the Heart Revisited. ISBN 978-94-010-7084-3
© 1988, Kluwer Academic Publishers, Dordrecht

is generally measured from the redevelopment of tension after shortening the muscle.[2,3] The effect of motion has not been tested under conditions where the influence of compliant regions extraneous to the cardiac sarcomere[4] can be ruled out. Not surprisingly, there is disagreement about its relevance to cardiac contraction, the role of 'activation', and most importantly, whether it reflects a property of the cross-bridge when and if it occurs.

Figure 1 shows experimental records of muscle length, force, and sarcomere length in an electrically stimulated, intact, isolated heart muscle preparation (source: rat, right ventricle). Peak shortening of the muscle clearly depends on its initial length even though the total load was kept constant (Figure 1A and 1B). The fact that peak shortening occurs at the same time here suggests that it is the initial length and/or the extent of motion which in some way influences the properties of the active muscle.

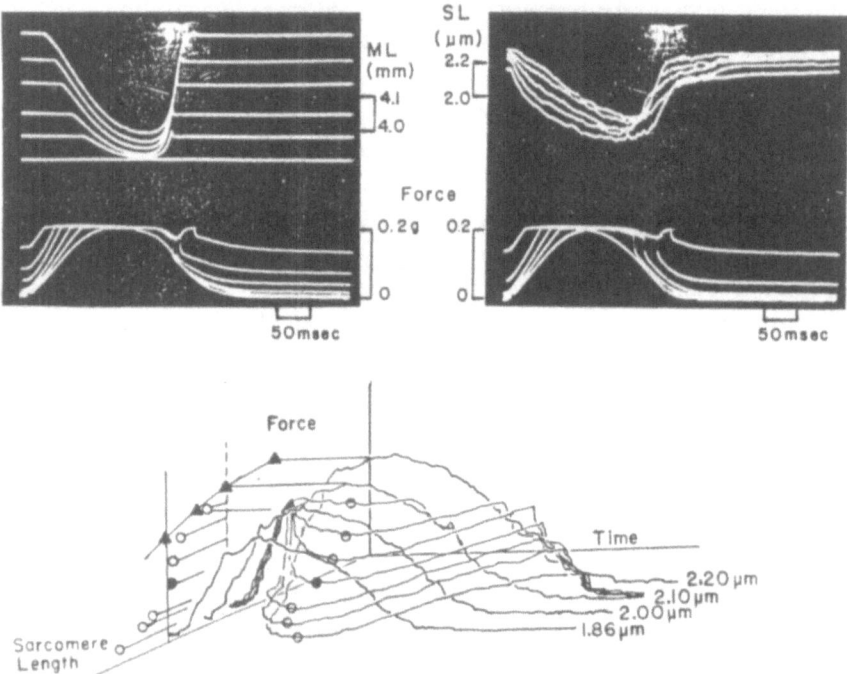

Fig. 1. The influence of initial length and/or motion on cardiac sarcomere shortening. The top photographs demonstrate the influence of initial length of the isolated muscle preparation (left) and of the sarcomere (right) in 5–6 contractions in which the total load was kept constant. The bottom most panel represents tracings from a computer-generated graphics display which compares the time course of isometric and isotonic contractions of the sarcomere. (The latter all start prior to peak contraction at a sarcomere length of 2.10 μms.) The filled triangles denote the projection of peak isometric tension on the force-length plane. The circles represent comparable projections at peak isotonic shortening. The sarcomeres do not shorten to that point expected from the dynamics of isometric tension development. This is shown by the vertical separation between the filled circle and the instantaneous isometric tension at SL = 1.86 μms.

Unfortunately, these possibilities become more difficult to evaluate when the time to peak shortening occurs after the peak of isometric contraction.[1] Actually, the full extent of sarcomere shortening will depend upon the dynamic surface defined by the rise and fall of its length-dependent ability to produce isometric force. This is illustrated best by a computerized, three-parameter display relating the influence of sarcomere length on isometric contraction. Such displays reveal that after the peak of contraction the sarcomere does not shorten isotonically to that point predicted by instantaneous isometric tension (Figure 1C). Importantly, this time corresponds to when the end points of cardiac ejection might occur.

While motion at the peak of contraction may depress contraction, the first phase of relaxation is also characterized by the decrease in isotonic shortening.[5,6] Therefore, we investigated the basic interaction between initial length and sarcomere motion at this time to learn whether these observations might reflect a common mechanism which limits cardiac muscle shortening.

Methods

Our experimental preparation is the right ventricular papillary or trabecular muscle, isolated from rat hearts. The muscles were electrically stimulated to contract 24/min in physiological solutions at 27°C. The light diffraction method, the experimental set up and solutions, and the statistical methods are described elsewhere.[4,5,6,7,8,9]

We first examined the effect of motion by varying the initial length in isotonic afterload contractions. Figure 2 shows how we defined the effect of shortening. The left hand panel gives a diagrammatic representation of the interrelations between sarcomere length and tension which occur in an isolated heart muscle preparation. Shortening occurs during the course of 12 isotonic contractions which start at different sarcomere lengths, ranging from 1.9 to 2.4 µms.

Due to the extraneous compliance in the isolated muscle preparation, internal shortening occurs auxotonically before the muscle preparation shortens isotonically. The isotonic point, SL_{iso}, occurs in time near when the myoplasmic calcium ion concentration is thought to peak and beyond which point it falls rapidly.[10] Figure 1B shows that SL_{iso} occurs earlier in contractions initiated at longer lengths, while the time at the end points of shortening is little affected. Since we wish to consider the effect of isotonic conditions alone, we consider only the influence of SL_{iso} upon the extent of net isotonic shortening, as shown at the right in Figure 2.

When prior motion and/or time do not influence contraction, the afterloaded muscle ought to shorten to the same end point, irrespective of initial

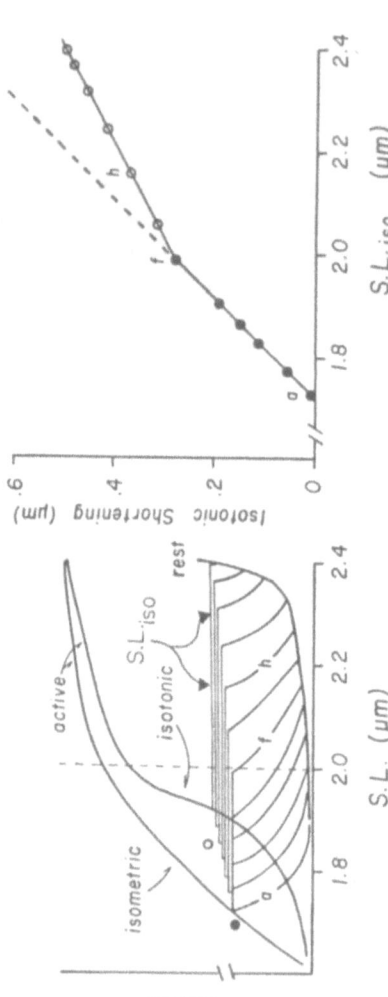

Fig. 2. One method of defining the effect of initial length upon isotonic motion in cardiac contraction. The left panel schematically shows the course of internal shortening in 12 afterloaded isotonic contractions which start from 12 different initial lengths. The bold outlines represent the endpoints of auxotonic and isotonic shortening is depicted in the right hand panel. The intercept with the abscissa denotes the point on the muscle's isometric length-tension relation (point 'a'). The slope of the initial length-total shortening relation will be less than one (dashed line) when an increase in initial length does not proportionately increment shortening (i.e., for $SL_{iso} > 2.0$ µms at 'f').

length. Consequently, any increase in shortening would equal the increment in SL_{iso}, and the corresponding relation between SL_{iso} and net isotonic shortening becomes a line with a slope equal to 1.0. However, shortening will cease at a longer length if motion depresses contractile activity. In this case, the increment in isotonic shortening will be less than the increment in initial length. Depression of contraction results in an isotonic shortening-initial length relation with a slope less than 1.0. (This is shown as points f and h, Fig. 2-right.)

For the moment, this diagram really presupposes our results. It simply illustrates a way of defining the effect of motion in the cardiac twitch. So far, there is no reason to expect that such simple linear relations really characterize the effect of motion length on contraction. But if true, the advantages of this approach are that: a) we can express the effect of shortening quantitatively by these slopes; b) it is not affected by the shape of the length-tension relation; and c) measurement of the effect of shortening does not require redevelopment of tension, so that any complications arising from a cooperative influence of cross-bridges[11] should be minimized. Finally, the method of analysis is more analogous to considering the determinants of ejection between the moment the aortic valve opens and closes.

Results

Effect of initial length

The above analysis of isotonic motion was devised and applied previously to the external dimensions of the isolated muscle preparation by Okada.[7] He plotted the afterloaded isotonic muscle shortening against its initial length. The relation for each load was found to be well described by a linear regression line with high statistical correlation. The slope of these relations decreased as the afterload was increased.[7] This behavior of the whole muscle was confirmed in our specimens as well, where these slopes were a) always less than one and b) also afterload-dependent.[8] In this respect, our results parallel specific findings of some previous studies[12,3,13] which also considered only external motions of the isolated muscle preparation.

However, in order to understand the basis for the effect of motion the length of the sarcomere must be measured. The dependence of isotonic shortening upon sarcomere length and afterload was then evaluated relative to SL_{iso}. Unlike the muscle, the full relation for the sarcomere shortening was best fit by two linear regression lines (Fig. 3). There was no deactivating effect at short sarcomere lengths; that is, the slope of the shortening relation was close to one and independent of load. At long sarcomere lengths,

48

however, the slope of the shortening relationship was again constant but always less than one. Here the slope decreased with an increase in load, as shown in Fig. 3. Also, like the findings for muscle shortening, an increase in activation (mediated by elevating extracellular calcium-reduced the depressant effect of an increase in initial length. The main difference is that when only the isotonic state of the muscle is considered, the positive impact on

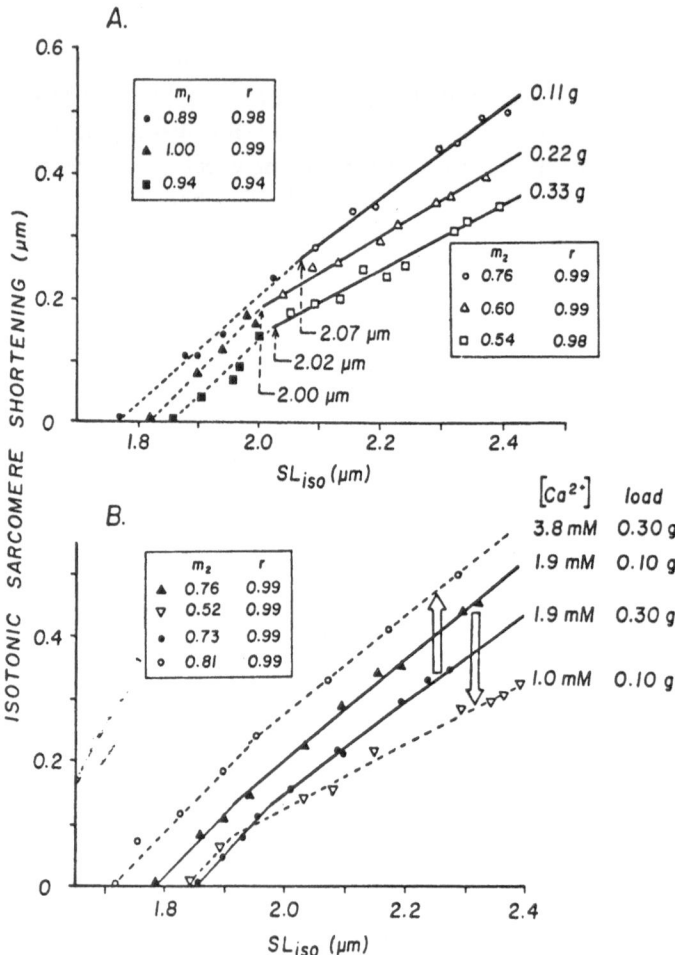

Fig. 3. Dependence of isotonic shortening of the sarcomere upon its initial length at the onset of isotonic conditions (SL$_{iso}$). (Top panel). m$_1$ and m$_2$ represent the slopes of the shortening relations when SL$_{iso}$ was less than or greater than 2.0 μms, respectively, and r represents the respective coefficients of linear regression. An effect of motion and afterload occurs only when SL$_{iso}$ > 2.0 μms at each afterload. (Bottom panel) The point of inflection between the two components of the shortening relation was not affected by inotropic state as caused by raising or lowering external calcium concentration (direction denoted by arrows). Figure adapted from Okada & Krueger.[9]

isotonic motion of lowering afterload or increasing activation have an additional effect which is confined to sarcomere lengths longer than 2.0 µms.

Both components of the length-isotonic shortening relationship were always well approximated by separate straight line fits of the data. Intriguingly, the sarcomere length at the inflection point was independent of load or inotropic state. The mean value for all 47 experiments was 2.00 ± 0.07 (SD) µms.[8,9] The effect of preload on shortening was identical in muscles which were allowed to shorten isotonically after a quick release or in those in which sarcomere length had been held constant before isotonic shortening. Limiting analysis to only the isotonic state of the muscle simply adjusts for internal auxotonic shortening. The early, undefined phase of contraction apparently does not alter the subsequent isotonic properties.

We also studied the motion effect with steady contraction using rapid cooling contractures which were initiated at different lengths and at constant afterload. (This method of activation is advantageous since the strength of steady contraction can be adjusted by changing external calcium.) As known from prior observations in muscle[14] and sarcomeres,[15] the effect of initial length was eliminated when activation is steady or high. Past differences in isotonic and isometric lengths[12,13] have been attributable to activation only in a nonspecific way. One interpretation of our data is that the depressive effect of shortening is not due to motion *per se* and it occurs only at long sarcomere lengths.

Controlled sarcomere shortening

One question is whether the distinct relation between initial length and shortening is a fortuitous result of our experimental design. Another kind of experiment is required to rule out the influence of time. The sarcomere was shortened at selected velocities by feedback control to a preselected length, starting *or* ending at a fixed moment during contraction. At a constant degree of sarcomere shortening, the re-development of tension was reduced when the preceding velocity of motion was high, as shown in Figs. 4A and B. Secondly, an increase in initial sarcomere length prior to shortening at a constant velocity decreases the development of tension both during and after controlled shortening (Fig. 4C). Comparable results have been described before in the external behavior of intact heart muscles.[3,16]

This kind of experiment rules out the influence of time. Moreover, comparison of the velocity dependence of, a) the slopes of the SL_{iso}-isotonic shortening relations (i.e., m_2 where $SL_{iso} > 2.0$ µms) and b) the deficit in isometric tension after controlled shortening, reveals an important difference (Fig. 4B). The depression of contraction by both methods is directly affected

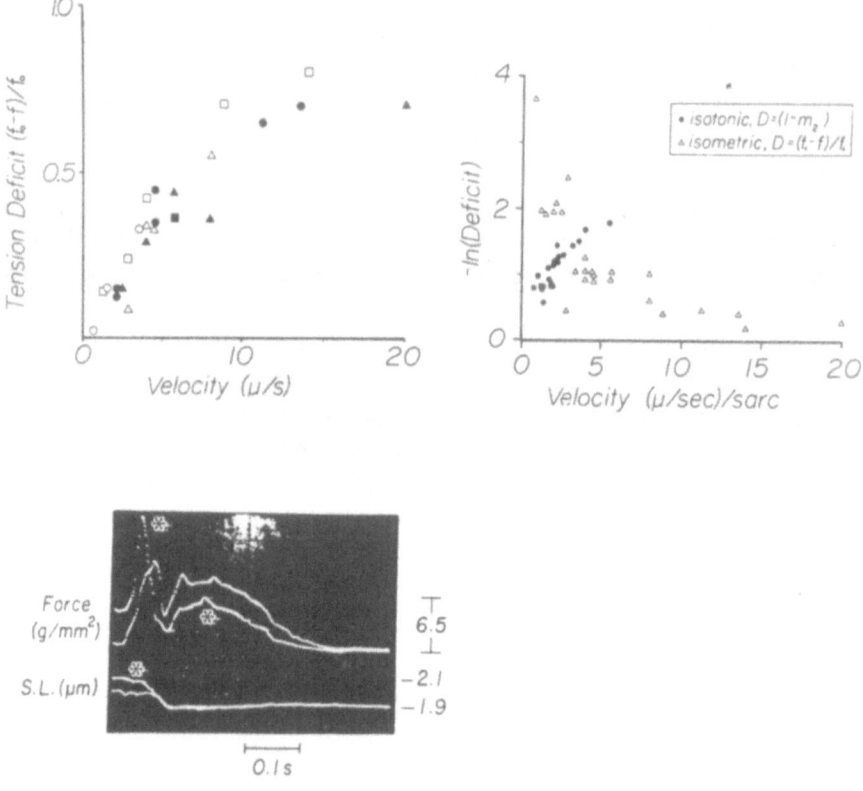

Fig. 4. Influence of controlled sarcomere motions upon the redevelopment of isometric tension. (Upper left panel) The deficit in redevelopment of tension after controlled sarcomere shortening of 0.2 μm at different velocities. The filled symbols denote onset of shortening at same time (0.1 sec, or 90% time to peak isometric tension), while the open symbols represent shortening completed at 0.1 sec. (Upper right panel) A comparison of the influence of velocity of motion on the depression of shortening $(1-m_2)$ and on the deficit in isometric tension development after controlled shortening. (Lower photograph) Like depression due to isotonic motion, an increase in the initial length and/or the extent of prior shortening decreases tension development at the same sarcomere length. Since depression of the respective modes of contraction differs with respect to the velocity of shortening, the effect of motion does not reside within the cross-bridge mechanism. Figure adapted from Okada & Krueger.[9]

by the extent of prior shortening, but each depends upon velocity in an opposite way. Thus, it is unlikely that the mechanism for the depression of isotonic motion resides within the turnover of the cross-bridge.

The length-dependent fall of isotonic shortening velocity

Cooperative interactions of the cross-bridge on calcium sensitivity[11] complicate interpretation of the effect of motion when tension is not constant as during and after controlled shortening. Therefore, we asked whether the dynamics of isotonic motions might account for the differences in the end points of sarcomere shortening?

Previous studies have not focussed on the early, length-dependent rapid fall of shortening velocity seen after a quick isotonic release. Rapid motions were thought to uncouple the contractile interactions (refer to Fig. 7[17]) since it was difficult to attribute explicitly the observations to the contractile element. However, an essential clue may reside in the manner in which the velocity slows with the sudden onset of isotonic shortening.

Figure 5 is a computerized display of the instantaneous dependence upon length of the velocity of sarcomere motion during contractions in which the muscle was quickly allowed to shorten isotonically near the peak of contraction. The sarcomeres had been first held isometric to prevent motion prior to the isotonic shortening. The velocity of sarcomere shortening was averaged over contiguous regions of the specimen, and then displayed as a function of instantaneous sarcomere length. A smooth line was then fitted to these curves, and the momentary dependence of velocity upon sarcomere length was then plotted as the logarithm of these values, as first suggested by Brenner[18] and shown in Figs. 5B and C.

Figure 5 reveals that the velocity of early shortening is proportional to sarcomere shortening when expressed in logarithmic coordinates. Moreover, the length-dependence of the early fall in velocity is independent of afterload. The precise shape and the underlying mechanisms which account for this fall in velocity are presently uncertain, but since the total load remains constant the dynamic effect of shortening can be considered analogous to an increase in the relative load on the sarcomere.

The length-dependent fall in the velocity of isotonic sarcomere shortening becomes more severe later in contraction as can be seen when the relative load is the same. Extrapolation of these relations back to the sarcomere length just prior to the isotonic release suggests that the rate of cross-bridge cycling a) changes little with activation but b) is more affected by shortening as time progresses.

Similar observations were first made by Brenner[18] who based his conclusions on measurements of the total length of directly activated papillary muscles. We show *here* that this behavior does indeed characterize the cardiac sarcomere in intact heart muscle. We further show that the peak, pre-release velocity does not change at those same times when we had previously measured a decrease in both 1) the maximum velocity of shortening (as extrapolated by the full, instantaneous force-velocity relations), and 2) the peak velocity of shortening in a quickly slackened muscle.[6]

Alternative ways exist for expressing the dynamic effect of shortening upon contraction, such as quantification of the curvature of the shortening traces

52

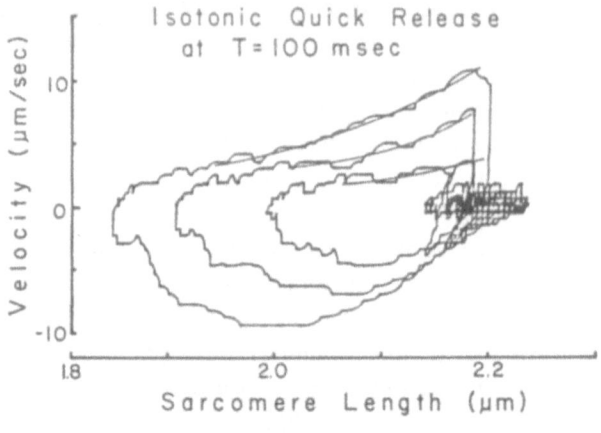

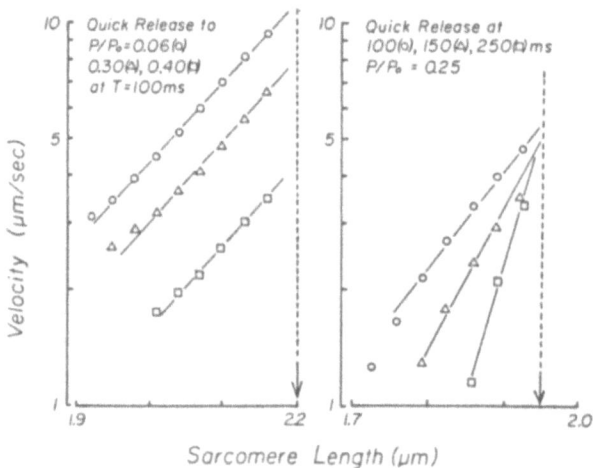

Sarcomere Length (μm)

Fig. 5. The dynamic influence of length on isotonic motions. (Top panel) The dependence of velocity upon sarcomere length after quick release to different isotonic tensions at the peak of contraction. Each trajectory represents the average of contiguous regions along the length of the preparation and where velocity was determined by a digital algorithm. (Lower left panel) The data in the upper panel was fit by a smooth curve and the fall of velocity in early shortening plotted in semilogarithmic form. The influence of shortening parallels that of an increase in afterload. (Lower right panel) The influence of isotonic motion upon the logarithmic velocity-length trajectory steepens when the sarcomeres are quickly shortened later in contraction. Extrapolation to the sarcomere length before the release (dashed line) indicates that after the peak of contraction the maximum rate of cross-bridge turnover is rapidly affected by shortening but not by time.

by fit to an exponential term with three constants. One advantage of the graphical method is that the influence of resting tension (when seen) can be evaluated and dismissed since the latter is readily visualized as an upward displacement from the semilogarithmic velocity-length trajectory.

How might motion and the sarcomere length at the onset of isotonic conditions interact to explain such an intrinsic effect of myofilament sliding Figure 6 shows that the initial fall in the velocity of isotonic shortening depends on sarcomere length. Paradoxically, at approximately the same moments (as denoted by horizontal lines) the velocity of shortening is the same at different sarcomere lengths. (At comparable times, we would have expected that the velocity to be higher at longer sarcomere lengths due to the steep sarcomere length-dependence of peak isometric force.)

The fall of velocity is not explained by statically determined length-dependent properties of the myofibrils since the steep length-dependence of maximum isometric tension at these levels of extracellular calcium (i.e., 1.9 mM) should have reduced the velocity at the shorter lengths accordingly. We would have expected the actual force on the shorter sarcomeres to be slightly greater at short lengths since resting tension is sustained in parallel to the cardiac sarcomere.[19] This effect should have additionally reduced the velocity of shortening, even though the total load remains constant.

Thus, the velocity of isotonic shortening appears to have been reduced by an increase in the length of the sarcomere at the onset of isotonic contraction. Finally, the data asymptotically approach the linear, parallel relation seen in the quick-release experiments. This is an indication that an effect of an increase in the initial length was similar to an increase in afterload seen in the isotonic quick releases. That is, the effective load on the shortening sarcomere is greater if its length was initially longer at the moment peak activation occurred.

Discussion

Initial length does not influence the end points of cardiac sarcomere shortening which occurs a) in the earliest phases of contraction, b) at very low loads, c) when sarcomere motion is auxotonic and when activation is high.[14,15,1,20] However, the mechanisms which completely govern shortening during the course of contraction are difficult to interpret when force changes[11]. Our observations demonstrate that a fundamental effect of initial length on isotonic shortening of the sarcomere occurs near the peak of contraction in isolated heart muscle. The effect, superimposed on the static properties of the myofibrils, would be most pronounced when shortening is slowed, the time of ejection is delayed, and activation is low as may occur in some cardiac diseases.[1]

We studied first the influence of active sarcomere length at the onset of isotonic shortening (SL_{iso}). At any afterload, the relationship between isotonic shortening and SL_{iso} was fitted well by two, discrete linear regression

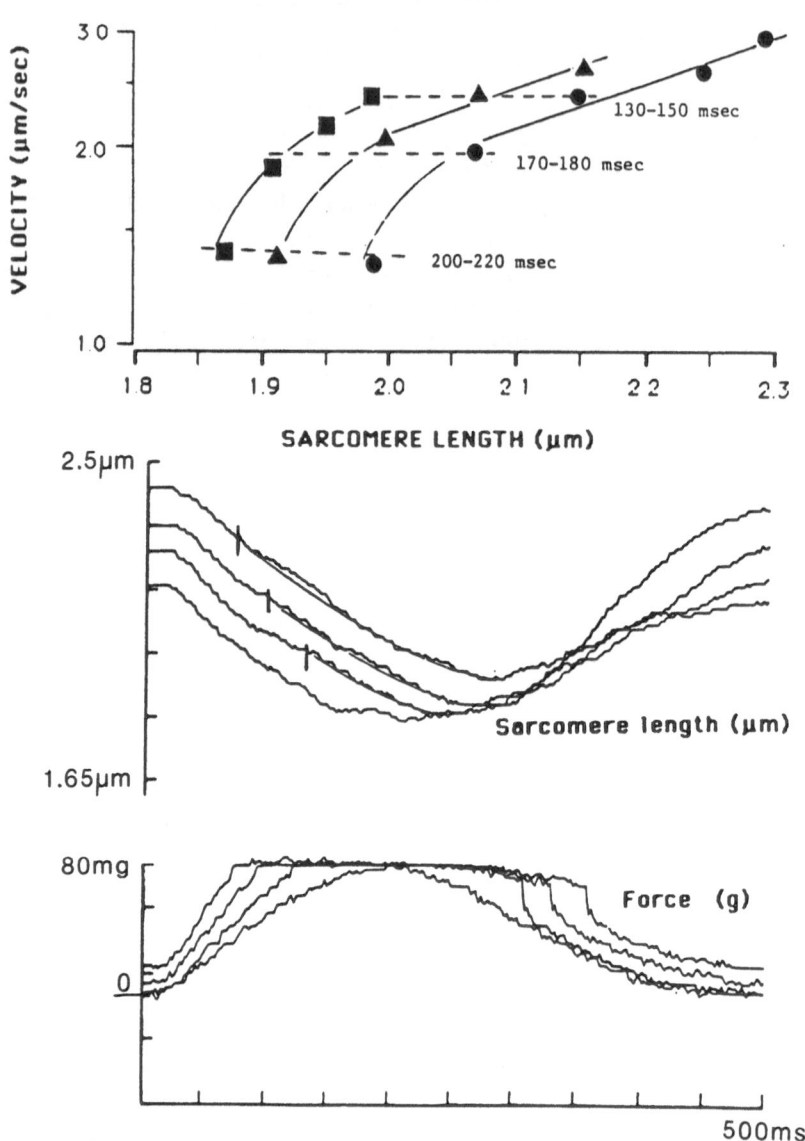

INFLUENCE OF PRELOAD ON AFTERLOADED
ISOTONIC VELOCITY TRAJECTORIES

Fig. 6. Influence of initial sarcomere length on the afterloaded isotonic velocity-length trajectories. The uppermost data point in each trajectory represents the sarcomere length at the onset of isotonic conditions (SL_{iso}). The lower panel shows the original data, where SL_{iso} is demarcated by vertical line. Shortening appears to reduce the dynamic properties of the sarcomere at these times in contraction.

lines of high correlation. This method showed that the end point of isotonic shortening is independent of initial length *unless* the sarcomere is longer than 2.0 μms at the *onset* of isotonic motion. The inflection where the slope of the SL_{iso}-shortening relation changes always occurred at a sarcomere length of 2.0 μms. Increases in force or decreases in external calcium concentration enhanced the influence of initial length on the end points of active shortening, but only in direct proportion to the original increment in SL_{iso} above 2.0 μms.[8,9]

We would not have expected such a simple relationship to characterize the complex interaction between length, force and time in isotonically shortening muscle. But as such, it provides a simple way to treat the variable influence of motion and load on ventricular function. Importantly, the isotonic method disregards the early phase of nonisotonic shortening and focusses upon the properties of the heart's muscle fibers *at the onset* of ejection.

The depression of shortening was directly related to the extent of isotonic motions occurring at $SL > 2.0$ μms. This parallels the effect of sarcomere shortening at constant velocity on the subsequent development of isometric tension. Depression of contraction in either case is related to the net translation of the myofilaments, but each depends in an opposite fashion upon the velocity of shortening. Thus, a mechanism confined to the cross-bridge cycle will not explain the depression of isotonic shortening. We found no evidence for an effect of motion at short lengths, and so the depression associated with isotonic motion cannot be due to deactivation or uncoupling of the contractile mechanism. The instantaneous relation between isotonic velocity and sarcomere length is smooth and continuous throughout the point of thin filament overlapping. Consequently, the deficit in the total isotonic shortening must reflect the initial conditions such as activation and/or sarcomere length. The velocity of shortening falls more rapidly than that predicted by an instantaneous length-dependence of activation of the myofibrils. The sarcomere length-dependence of velocity shows that the instantaneous effect of isotonic shortening resembles the effect of an increase in load on the sarcomere. Intriguingly, these length-dependent features of the contractile dynamics are established relatively early in contraction, but predominate at the peak of contraction where the end points of ejection occur. For example, we can calculate from Figure 5B that the dynamic load-displacement of the velocity trajectory is equivalent to $\sim 0.16P/0.1$ μm, where P is isometric tension. It is provocative that a 'full load'-velocity displacement (i.e., $[Pmax/0.16P] \times 0.1$ μm $= 0.6$ μm) completely spans the functional range of sarcomere shortening[15,20]...even though the former parameter is measured in the early phases of shortening. (Moreover, the effect of an increment in initial sarcomere length of 0.1 μm in the controlled shortening (Fig. 4C) was to reduce the redevelopment of isometric force by approximately 1/6 of the maximum.) Thus, the dynamics of early shortening parallel the effect of length on the end points of isotonic shortening.

The linear dependence of net isotonic shortening upon SL_{iso} and the occurrence of an inflection point at 2.0 µms suggest that initial conditions affect the end points of contraction. Moreover, the instantaneous influence of length on the dynamics of shortening suggests that the effect of isotonic motion is equivalent to an increase in the internal load in the shortening sarcomere. For the moment, both can be explained if length and tension interact to influence the *distribution* of activation along the thin filament.

Hypothesis – end effects

The linearity of the isotonic shortening relations suggests a simple model in which initial sarcomere length, the number of cross-bridges, and myofibrillar calcium binding interact to alter the distribution of active sites on the filament. Consider, for example, a case where the part of the thin filament in the I band would be less activated because of the absence of cross-bridges (Fig. 7). (Alternatively, dissociation of calcium from the thin filaments could occur first in the I-band.) When the sarcomere now shortens, the less activated parts of the thin filament would enter the A-band. Since the cytosolic calcium transient declines very quickly, these relatively unactivated parts would not proportionately increment tension development. Thus, motion would be misconstrued as depressing the contractile interactions. The effect of initial length would disappear at a sarcomere length of 2.0 µms if a) there are elements at the ends of the sarcomere which locally compete with the regulatory proteins for calcium binding or if b) a region of the thin filament which is most accessible to changing levels of cytoplasmic calcium is exposed only at long sarcomere lengths. The microscopic appearance of the striation pattern in isolated heart cells[19] and the steep shape of the cardiac length tension relation can also be interpreted in terms of lack of activation at the ends of the shortened sarcomere.

The existence of length-dependent, longitudinal gradients of activation can explain all of our results and leads to some testable predictions. Firstly, when the sarcomere shortens isotonically, the load on the cross-bridges would increase as the inactivated region of the thin filament enters the A-band, thereby restricting the sites for cross-bridge formation. Thus, specific conditions would exist when the rate of tension fall would be constant and proportional to sarcomere shortening at a constant velocity.[18,21] Secondly, sarcomeres isotonically shortened from longer initial lengths should be weaker and therefore relengthen to respectively longer lengths when pulled upon by a sudden increase in isotonic load. Conversely, our model would be

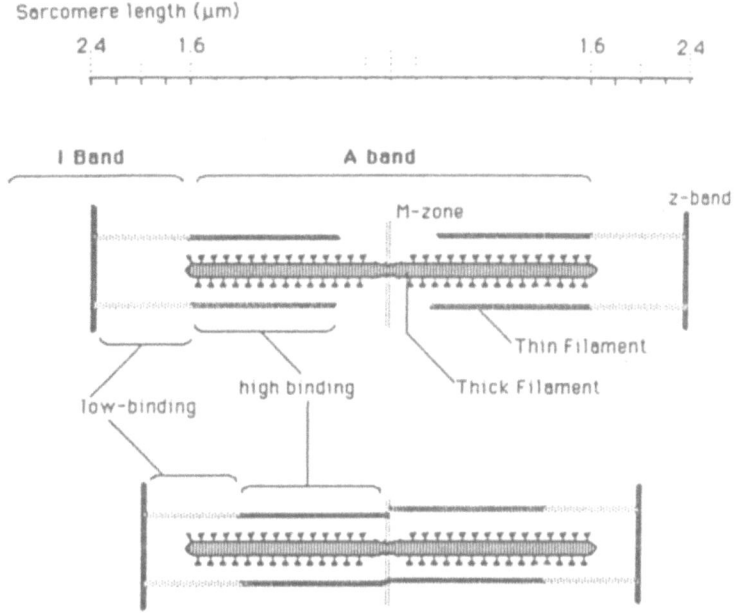

Sorcomere length (μm)

2.4   1.6   1.6   2.4

I Band   A band   z-band

M-zone

Thin Filament

high binding   Thick Filament

low-binding

ISOTONICALLY SHORTENED SARCOMERE

Fig. 7. A simple model in which initial sarcomere length, the number of cross-bridges in the overlap-zone, and calcium binding interact to alter the distribution of active sites on the thin filament. Since intracellular calcium transient declines very quickly, the relatively inactivated portion originally in the I-band would not promote tension development when the sarcomere shortens at and after the peak of contraction. This would increase the relative load on the cross-bridges even though total load remains constant on the sarcomere, thereby inhibiting shortening beyond that predicted by the instantaneous effect of length on purely isometric tension. In this way, an End Effect due to the length of the I-band might influence the subsequent dynamic properties of heart muscle.

refuted if the fall of the cytoplasmic calcium transient were to be altered when net isotonic shortening was increased by increments in initial length. This effect is opposite to fall of calcium transient when shortening is promoted by decreases in afterload.[10]

Our working model assumes that an effect of initial length arises from lack of cross-bridge formation in the end region (An 'I-band' Effect). The effect of initial length would be much larger if cross-bridges attach but 'stick', thereby creating a drag within the inactivated region. This form of 'End Effect' would always be proportional to increments in initial length and, unlike an I-band Effect, be independent of sarcomere length throughout the full range of myofilament overlap.

By our definition, an End Effect represents an influence of motion on contraction which occurs at long sarcomere lengths. This situation constitutes

58

a positive feedback mechanism when initial sarcomere length is $>2.0\,\mu$ms which would augment 'end diastolic length' when a fixed relengthening is enforced after an increment in afterload. Thus, an End Effect predicts an equilibrium between activation and secondary adjustments in end diastolic volume when cardiac filling is made constant. This mechanism links depressed activation with lowered cardiac function.

Finally, an inactive region at the ends of the sarcomere, established by the time of onset of isotonic motion, can explain how the nature of loading and initial length might interact to variably influence the contractile performance of the heart. For the moment, a simple model suggests that an effect of shortening on contraction does not have to be a direct property of the cross-bridges or of the statically determined properties of the myofibril.

Acknowledgements

This work was supported, in part, by a NIH grant in aid HL 21325 and an Established Fellowship from the New York Heart Association (JK) and a Fellowship from the Japan Society for the Promotion of Science (TO).

References

1. Strobeck JE, Krueger JW and Sonnenblick EH (1980). Load and time considerations in the force-length relation of cardiac muscle. Fed Proc 39: 45–52.
2. Edman KAP (1975). Mechanical deactivation induced by shortening in isolated muscle fibers of the frog. J Physiol 246: 255–275.
3. Leach JK, Brady AJ, Skipper BJ and Mills DL (1980). Effects of active shortening on tension development of rabbit papillary muscle. Am J Physiol 238: H8–H13.
4. Krueger JW and Pollack GH (1975). Myocardial sarcomere dynamics during isometric contraction. J Physiol 251: 627–643.
5. Krueger JW and Farber S (1980). Sarcomere length 'orders' relaxation in cardiac muscle. Eur Heart J 1 (Suppl A): 37–47.
6. Krueger JW and Tsujioka K (1982). Sarcomere relaxation mechanisms in isolated heart muscle. Biophys J 37: 360a.
7. Okada T (1980). Depressive effect of active shortening on stroke volume of left ventricle and shortening amount of isolated ventricular muscle. Jpn J Physiol 31: 199–215.
8. Okada T, Glassman R and Krueger JW (1983). Shortening deactivation depends on sarcomere length in isolated rat heart muscle. Circulation 68: III–417.
9. Okada T and Krueger JW (1985). A depressant effect of shortening depends on sarcomere length in isolated heart muscle. (Submitted).
10. Housmans PR, Lee NKM and Blinks JR (1983). Active shortening retards the decline of the intracellular calcium transient in mammalian heart muscle. Science 221: 159–161.
11. Bremel RD and Weber A (1972). Cooperations within actin filaments in vertebrate skeletal muscle. Nature New Biol 238: 97–101.
12. Brady AJ (1967). Length-tension relations in cardiac muscle. Am Zool 7: 603–610.
13. Taylor RR (1970). Active length-tension relations compared in isometric and isotonic contractions of cat papillary muscle. Circ Res 26: 279–288.

14. Downing SE and Sonnenblick EH (1964). Cardiac muscle mechanics and ventricular performance: force and time parameters. Am J Physiol 207: 705–715.
15. Pollack GH and Krueger JW (1976). Sarcomere dynamics in intact cardiac muscle. Eur J Cardiol 4 Suppl: 53–65.
16. Meiss RA and Sonnenblick EH (1972). Controlled shortening in heart muscle: Velocity-force and active state properties. Am J Physiol 222: 630–639.
17. Brutsaert DL and Sonnenblick EH (1969). Force-velocity-length-time relations of the contractile elements in heart muscle of the cat. Circ Res 24: 137–149.
18. Brenner B (1980). Effect of free sarcoplasmic Ca^{2+} concentration on maximum unloaded shortening velocity: measurements on single glycerinated rabbit psoas muscle fibres. J Mus Res Cell Mot 1: 409–428.
19. Krueger JW and London B (1984). Contraction bands: Differences between physiologically vs. Maximally activated single heart muscle cells. Adv Exp Med Biol 170: 119–134.
20. ter Keurs HEDJ, Rijnsburger WH, van Heuningen R and Negelsmit MJ (1980). Tension development and sarcomere length in rat cardiac trabeculae: evidence of length-dependent activation. Circ Res 46: 703–714.
21. Brenner B and Jacob R (1980). Calcium activation and maximum unloaded shortening velocity. Investigations on glycerinated skeletal and heart muscles preparations. Basic Res Cardiol 75: 40–46.

5. The Relation Between Contraction Dynamics and the Intracellular Calcium Transient in Mammalian Cardiac Muscle

PHILIPPE R. HOUSMANS

Department of Anesthesiology, Mayo Foundation, Rochester, Minnesota, USA

Contraction dynamics and intracellular calcium

The contraction of cardiac muscle is the end result of several steps that constitute excitation–contraction coupling: action potential, entry of Ca^{2+} ions through the surface membrane, release of Ca^{2+} ions from intracellular stores (sarcoplasmic reticulum), binding of Ca^{2+} to the C subunit of the regulatory protein troponin on the thin filament, conformational changes in the thin filament to uncover the myosin binding sites on actin molecules, the binding of myosin heads of actin through the formation of myosin cross-bridges, and finally, motion of cross-bridges that result in force development and/or shortening. The detailed study of each of the above mentioned steps has become almost a field of investigation of its own. There is increasing evidence for the existence of several feedback loops between steps in excitation–contraction coupling, of which only a few will be mentioned in this chapter. Mechanical events such as changes in length alter the characteristics of both the action potential[1-4] and of the intracellular Ca^{2+} transient[4-7] detected with the Ca^{2+}-regulated photoprotein aequorin[8]. The purpose of this brief review is to highlight the observations that changes in load or of force development influence the time course of the intracellular calcium transient in isolated cardiac muscle. It will become apparent that it is often not possible to distinguish between changes of length and of force as the *primum movens* for the observed changes in the intracellular calcium transient.

1. *The phenomenon of "shortening deactivation"*

In many kinds of striated muscle, the terminal or isometric phase of relaxation proceeds at earlier times when the muscle is allowed to shorten during a twitch than when it was constrained to contract isometrically

H.E.D.J. ter Keurs and M.I.M. Noble (eds), Starling's Law of the Heart Revisited. ISBN 978-94-010-7084-3
© 1988, Kluwer Academic Publishers, Dordrecht

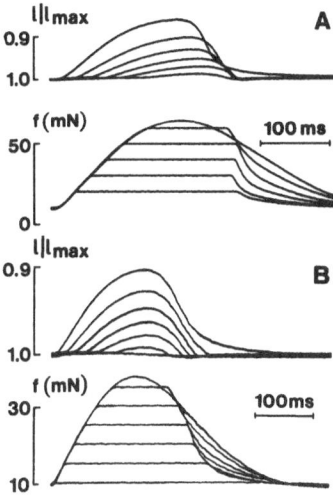

Fig. 1. Shortening deactivation or load-sensitivity of relaxation in mammalian ventricular muscle. Temperature 30 C, stimulus interval 5 seconds, $[Ca^{2+}]$ 2.5 mM.

Panel A: Length (upper) and force (lower) traces of an isometric and of five afterloaded isotonic twitches of a right ventricular cat papillary muscle were superimposed. Whenever shortening occurred during the twitch, isometric relaxation fell short in time of that of the isometric control twitch.

Panel B: Same format as in panel A. Shortening deactivation in rat left ventricular papillary muscle.

throughout. This typical dissociation of force traces in isometric relaxation is found in ventricular muscle of cats,[9] ferrets,[10] rats,[9,11–13] pigs,[9] and in many kinds of skeletal muscle[14,15] (Fig. 1). This phenomenon has commonly been referred to as "shortening deactivation". In comparison with isometric contractions, in lightly loaded contractions, muscle shortening is associated with a prolonged depolarization and a prolongation of the action potential,[2,3] as well as with a slowing of the decline of the intracellular calcium transient[5,6] yet without any apparent prolongation of the total duration of the Ca^{2+} transient. This has been shown for isolated right ventricular papillary muscle of the cats,[5,6] ferret (Fig. 2), in frog ventricular strips (unpublished observations). Furthermore, the observation that muscle shortening causes the same change of the calcium transients during twitch contractions of single fibers of the frog tibialis anterior[7]. This is important to refute the consideration that with the use of multicellular preparations (such as papillary muscles and trabeculae), aequorin signals may not be truly representative of those cells that participate in the contractile events of muscle, as aequorin signals originate from injected superficial cells only. The mechanical change, i.e. the onset of shortening, preceded the extra "light of shortening" by some 35 milliseconds in the cat papillary muscle at 30 C[6]. Conversely, when in a

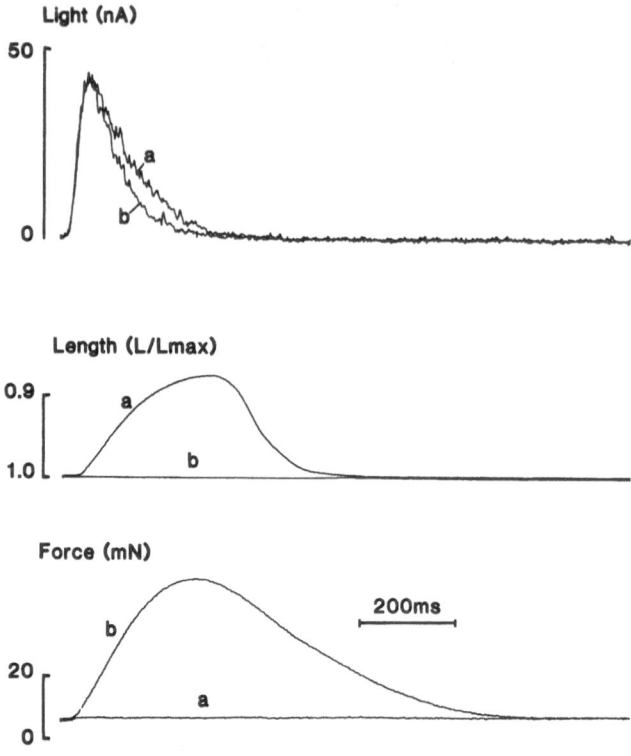

Fig. 2. Light emission by aequorin (upper), length (middle), and force (lower) traces of an isotonic preloaded (a) twitch and an isometric twitch (b) of ferret right ventricular papillary muscle. Both contractions were preceded by an equal number of isometric twitches at the initial muscle length L_{max}. Shortening (a) is associated with a slower decline of the intracellular calcium transient ("light of shortening"). Stimulus interval 4 seconds, 30 C, $[Ca^{2+}]$ 2.25 mM. Eight contractions were averaged to improve the signal-to-ratio. Light was recorded with a time constant of 1 ms.

lightly loaded twitch contraction, muscle shortening was stopped in mid-course, and muscles were forced to continue contraction in the isometric mode at that shorter length, light emission by aequorin decreased in comparison with twitches where shortening had not been stopped in mid-course.[6]

The changes of intracellular Ca^{2+} concentration followed the mechanical change by some 30–50 milliseconds (at 30 C). Similar maneuvers of shortening are known to cause a small depolarization of the cell membrane[4] and a prolongation of the action potential.[2–4] However, since in a given contraction the changes in myoplasmic $[Ca^{2+}]_i$ associated with shortening precede rather than follow the changes in the transmembrane potential, it is likely that the changes of $[Ca^{2+}]_i$ are the cause rather than effects of the changes in the action potential. Allen et al. have subsequently demonstrated that the increase of light emission by aequorin after a quick release in the cat papillary muscle preceded shortening-induced depolarization of the cell membrane by some 20 milliseconds at 30 C.[4] The increase in $[Ca^{2+}]_i$ leads to a positive change in the membrane potential, possibly by activation of an electrogenic Na^+-Ca^{2+} exchange perhaps combined with opening of nonspecific channels which carry Na^+ and K^+ ions. [4]

2. Mechanism for the increased $[Ca^{2+}]_i$ associated with shortening

There is considerable evidence that the increase in myoplasmic Ca^{2+} concentrations with shortening (or the associated lack of force development) relative to that during force development is due to less calcium being bound or to calcium being released from contractile filaments (more specifically, troponin C, since this is the calcium-binding protein of most significant interest in cardiac contraction) as a consequence of a diminished affinity of troponin C for calcium resulting from a decrease in the number of cross-bridges during a period of shortening.[1,16] The biochemical basis for this argument was first suggested by Bremel and Weber,[17] who showed that the formation of rigor myosin cross-bridges increased the affinity for Ca^{2+} of the low-affinity sites of troponin C, a feature that may be true for cross-bridges during their normal cycling mode as well (for references see 18). Allowing a muscle to shorten would then decrease the affinity of troponin C for Ca^{2+} so that less Ca^{2+} will be bound to troponin C after a period of shortening than after a comparable period of force development. Since in mammalian cardiac muscle the calcium cannot be regained by troponin C and rapid relaxation (lengthening) follows. According to this hypothesis, more calcium will be bound at the peak of the isometric twitch, and less calcium is required to maintain continued cross-bridge interaction during the slow isometric relaxation. This hypothesis can therefore account for the phenomenon of "shortening deactivation" or "load-sensitivity of relaxation".[9] There is abundant experimental evidence from studies both in skinned and intact muscle fibers that muscle length affects the calcium responsiveness of the contractile proteins, most likely the affinity of troponin C for Ca^{2+} (reviewed in ref. 1). Yet, as noted earlier, it is difficult in most instances to dissociate effects of length *per se* from effects of load, force development, or lack thereof during shortening on the increase in $[Ca^{2+}]_i$ seen during a quick release where both length and force are changing, the latter being a function of the number of cross-bridges. Is the Ca^{2+} bound to troponin C then a function of length, or of the number of cross-bridges (force), or both In at least two circumstances it has been possible to infer the role of force on the light emission by aequorin in shortening muscle. First, in the cat papillary muscle, the increase in light associated with shortening over a limited range (less than 10% of L_{max})

against a constant load was larger than any difference in light seen in isometric twitches at those two different lengths.[6] Second, in skinned ferret papillary muscle[19] a 10% decrease in length during contracture in a low Ca^{2+} (~ 15 M) environment caused both an abrupt drop in force and a rise in light emission by aequorin, both of which occurred almost simultaneously. Upon stretching the muscle back to its initial length, muscle force returned in two phases: a fast increase and a much slower increase. The decrease of light emission by aequorin was gradual and seemed temporally better related to the changes of force than to those of length. These observations have also rendered less likely the possibility that the extra Ca^{2+} seen during shortening comes from a membranous compartment. Hofmann and Fuchs reported that in detergent extracted bovine ventricular bundles (where troponin C was the only calcium-binding species) the binding of Ca^{2+} to cardiac troponin C was length dependent but that this length dependence disappeared when rigor cross-bridge formation was suppressed in the presence of vanadate.[20] They concluded that length dependence of the binding of calcium to troponin C is dependent on the formation of cross-bridges, a hypothesis that is compatible with biochemical data showing that rigor bond formation increased the affinity of troponin C for Ca^{2+}.[17] In addition, when the binding of Ca^{2+} was measured during ATP-induced force generation and during vanadate-induced relaxation over the same pCa range, force-generating fibers bound more Ca^{2+} than the vanadate-relaxed fibers.[21] Yet, in Triton X-100 skinned canine cardiac fibers, Pan and Solaro[22] found little difference in Ca^+-binding properties of troponin C between fibers contracting freely and those generating force while contracting isometrically, suggesting that the number of attached cross-bridges has little impact on troponin C. Reasons for this discrepancy are not clear, yet if the number of cross-bridges attached at any time during normal cycling is small, the alteration of overall Ca^{2+} affinity of troponin C may be too small to resolve.[22] Finally, in addition to cooperativity in thin filament activation due to cross-bridge formation, there is compelling evidence in skeletal muscle for longitudinal cooperativity of Ca^{2+} binding within the thin filament due to long-range interactions possibly involving tropomyosin as the transducing element.[23] It has recently become apparent that myocardial contractility is also subject to regulation by muscle length *between* contractions. Short muscle lengths during the diastolic interval between isometric twitches produces a negative inotropic effect that is proportional to the time spent at the shorter length.[24] Length-sensitivity of Ca^{2+} entry[24] or extrusion mechanisms[25] and/or length-sensitivity of Ca^{2+} release or uptake by the sarcoplasmic reticulum[25] seem possible mechanisms, but at present this issue has not been settled.

3. *Influence of load over several contractions*

It is a well-known phenomenon in mammalian cardiac muscle that the mode of contraction (isometric versus isotonic) influences the amplitude of contraction in subsequent twitches.[2,26-28] In the cat papillary muscle, the first isometric twitch after a series of at least seven isotonic twitches against preload only, has a higher peak amplitude than the second and subsequent isometric twitches, until a steady state is reached after seven to eight twitches. Conversely, when the mode of contraction is switched from isometric to isotonic between contractions, the first isotonic twitch after a series of isometric twitches is smaller than the next isotonic, and a new steady state is reached after four to eight contractions. When, after a series of stable isometric twitches (stimulus interval 4 seconds, 30 C), muscles were allowed to shorten isotonically from the same initial length, the amplitude of the aequorin signal (peak light) increased in successive twitches, herewith paralleling the increase in the amplitude of contraction.[28] The peak of the of the aequorin signal in the first isotonic twitch was of the same amplitude as in the immediately preceding isometric twitch; yet the decline of the aequorin signal was slower in this and all succeeding isotonic twitches. It is conceivable that an increased intracellular calcium availability builds up in successive isotonic contractions, as the native Ca^{2+}-affinity of troponin C is less than during force development and leads to more releasable Ca^{2+} from intracellular stores in subsequent twitches. At higher frequencies of stimulation or lower temperatures, all changes were attenuated or even reversed.[28-30]

Support: USPHS International Research Fellowship TW03046 and grants HL12186 and GM36365.

References

1. Allen DG and Kentish JC (1985). The cellular basis of the length–tension relation in cardiac muscle. J Mol Cell Cardiol 17: 821–840.
2. Kaufmann RL, Lab MJ, Hennekes R and Krause H (1971). Feedback interaction of mechanical and electrical events in the isolated mammalian ventricular myocardium (cat papillary muscle). Pflugers Arch 324: 100–123.
3. Hennekes R, Kaufmann RL and Lab MJ (1981). The dependence of cardiac membrane excitation and contractile activity on active muscle shortening (cat papillary muscle). Pflugers Arch 392: 22–28.
4. Lab MJ, Allen DG and Orchard CH (1984). The effects of shortening on myoplasmic calcium concentration and on the action potential in mammalian ventricular muscle. Circ Res 55: 825–829.
5. Allen DG, Cannell MB, Lab JM and Orchard CH (1983). Shortening during contraction slows the calcium transient in cat papillary muscle. J Physiol (London) 334: 108P–109P.
6. Housmans PR, Lee NKM and Blinks JR (1983). Active shortening retards the decline of the intracellular calcium transient in mammalian heart muscle. Science 217: 159–161.

66

7. Blinks JR, Lee NKM and Housmans PR (1983). Shortening deactivation in frog skeletal muscle is not associated with abbreviation of the intracellular calcium transient. Fed Proc 42: 569.

8. Blinks JR, Wier WG, Hess P and Prendergast FG (1982). Measurements of Ca^{2+} concentrations in living cells. Prog Biophys Mol Biol 40: 1–114.

9. Brutsaert DL, Housmans PR and Goethals MA (1980). Its role in the ventricular function in the mammalian heart. Circ Res 47: 637–652.

10. Housmans PR and Murat I. Comparative effects of halothane, enflurane, and isoflurane at equipotent anesthetic doses on isolated ventricular myocardium of the ferret. Anesthesiology (in press).

11. Poggesi C, Reggiani C, Ricciardi L and Minelli R (1982). Factors modulating the sensitivity of the relaxation to the loading conditions in rat cardiac muscle. Pflugers Arch 394: 338–346.

12. Poggesi C, Reggiani C, Bottinelli R, Ricciardi L and Minelli R (1983). Relaxation in atrial and ventricular myocardium: activation decay and different load-sensitivity. Basic Res Cardiol 78: 256–265.

13. Lecarpentier YC, Chuck LHS, Housmans PR, De Clerck NM and Brutsaert DL (1979). Nature of load dependence of relaxation in cardiac muscle. Am J Physiol 237: H455–H460.

14. Jewell BR and Wilkie DR (1960). The mechanical properties of relaxing muscle. J Physiol (London) 152: 30–47.

15. Bahler AS (1971). Mechanical properties of relaxing frog skeletal muscle. Am J Physiol 220: 1983–1990.

16. Ridgway EB and Gordon AM (1984). Muscle calcium transient: effects of poststimulus length changes in single fibers. J Gen Physiol 83: 75–103.

17. Bremel RD and Weber A (1972). Cooperation within actin filaments in vertebrate skeletal muscle. Nature PBbBbPNew Biology 238: 97–101.

18. Blinks JR and Endoh M (1986). Modification of myofibrillar responsiveness to Ca^{2+} as an inotropic mechanism. Circulation 73 (Suppl III): 85–97.

19. Allen DG and Kentish JC (1985). The effects of length changes on the myoplasmic calcium concentration in skinned ferret ventricular muscle. J Physiol (London) 336: 67P.

20. Hofmann PA and Fuchs F (1985). Effect of length and cross–bridge attachment on Ca^{2+} binding to cardiac troponin C. Am J Physiol 253: C90–C96.

21. Hofmann PA and Fuchs F (1986). Evidence for a force dependent component of Ca^{2+} binding to cardiac troponin C. Biophys J 49: 84.

22. Pan BS and Solaro RJ (1987). Calcium-binding properties of troponin C in detergent-skinned heart muscle fibers. J Biol Chem 262: 7839–7849.

23. Moss RL, Allen JD and Greaser ML (1986). Effects of partial extraction of troponin complex upon the tension-pCa relation in rabbit skeletal muscle. Further evidence that tension development involves cooperative effects within the thin filament. J Gen Physiol 87: 761–774.

24. Nichols CG (1985). The influence of 'diastolic' length on the contractility of isolated cat papillary muscle. J Physiol (London) 361: 269–279.

25. Hanck DA and Jewell BR (1985). Effects of physiological beating on the contractility of cat ventricular muscle. Am J Physiol 248: H894–H900.

26. Parmley WW, Brutsaert DL and Sonnenblick EH (1969). Effects of altered loading on contractile events in isolated cat papillary muscle. Circ Res 24: 521–532.

27. Jewell BR and Rovell JM (1973). Influence of previous mechanical events on the contractility of isolated cat papillary muscle. J Physiol (London) 235: 715–740.

28. Housmans PR, Lee NKM and Blinks JR (1983). History of loading in preceding contractions influences intracellular calcium transients in the cat papillary muscle. Fed Proc 42: 573.

29. Donald TC, Peterson DM, Walker AA and Hefner LL (1976). Afterload-induced homeometric autoregulation in isolted cardaic muscle. Am J Physiol 231: 545–550.

30. Wahler GM, Swayze CR and Fox IJ (1984). A Ca^{2+}-dependent mechanism for the positive inotropic response to an increase in afterload in cat papillary muscle. Can J Physiol Pharmacol 62: 296–301.

6. The Effects of Sarcomere Length on Force and Velocity of Shortening in Cardiac Muscle

H.E.D.J. TER KEURS, B. WOHLFART, L. RICCIARDI & J.J.J. BUCX

Department of Physiology, The Faculty of Medicine, The University of Calgary, Calgary, Alberta, Canada

Abstract

The relation between peak force (F) during contraction, velocity of shortening (V) and sarcomere length (SL) determine cardiac pump function. We have studied the factors that control force and velocity of shortening were studied in trabeculae dissected from normal or hypertrophied right ventricles of rats in modified Krebs-Henseleit solution at 26 C, in which Ca^{2+} or pH was varied. Hypertrophy (H) was induced by triiodothyronine injections (Ht), by vigorous physical exercise during swimming (Hs) or by hypobaric hypoxia (Hh).

The relation between F and SL was convex toward the F axis at $Ca^{2+} > 0.5$ mM, linear at $Ca^{2+} = 0.5$ mM, and convex toward the SL axis at $Ca^{2+} < 0.5$ mM. The shape of the F–SL relations varied with pH in a similar manner as with Ca^{2+}.

V closely approximated a rectangular hyperbolic function of F: $V(F + a) = b(F_o - F)$ under all conditions ($F_o =$ maximal F at the SL at which the relation is studied). $a = 9.52 \pm 5.6$ mM/mm^2, $b = 1.00 \pm 0.45$ mm/ s and $V_o = 13.6 \pm 3.0$ µm/s in controls (C) ($V_o = V$ at $F = 0$ and $SL = 2.00$ µm). The hyperbolic relationship fitted the data also during stretch of the sarcomeres at velocities that approached 1 µm/s, at which F increased up to $4 \times F_o$.

V_o was constant under all conditions in which developed Force exceeded 40% F at a $SL = 2.00$ µm at $Ca^{++} = 2.5$ mM: 1) V_o was independent of SL at $SL > 1.85$ µm; 2) V_o increased during the twitch to a maximum at 25 ms following the start and then remained constant up to 100 ms thereafter; 3) V_o increased with increasing Ca_o^{++} and reached maximal values at Ca_o^{2+} above 1.0 mM; 4) V_o was constant at pH > 6.7. V_o, furthermore, increased in the order Hh, C, Hs, Ht, corresponding to an increase of the myosin ATPase activity and to the shift of the myosin isoenzyme distribution under these conditions.

H.E.D.J. ter Keurs and M.I.M. Noble (eds), Starling's Law of the Heart Revisited. ISBN 978-94-010-7084-3

This observed behaviour of the F–SL relation is consistent with the hypothesis that the F–SL relations are determined by length-dependent sensitivity of the contractile system to calcium, while protons seem to compete with calcium ions in a length-independent fashion. The behaviour of V_o can be explained if V_o is sensitive to the amount of calcium that is bound to the contractile proteins. V_o, therefore, depends on the level of activation and as a result of length dependent sensitivity of the contractile apparatus on sarcomere length.

Introduction

Force development of cardiac muscle increases with increasing sarcomere length and varied Ca_o^{2+}.[1] Studies of the mechanism(s) underlying length dependence of force development addressed in Chapter 1 suggest that length controls the sensitivity of the contractile system to calcium ions thereby controls the number of active force generators.

Length dependence of velocity of shortening has been shown as well, both in shortening velocity of overall length of cardiac muscle of cat,[2] segment shortening as measured by recording the cross sectional area of the papillary muscle of Ferret[3] and sarcomere shortening of trabeculae of Rat measured by light diffraction techniques.[1] The relation between velocity of shortening and length differed from the way in which force depends on length. The mechanism of length dependence of Vo is unclear particularly as it has been observed over a length range in which internal passive forces in the muscle are negligible.[4,5] One wonders, therefore, if an alternative explanation can be found in dependence of the maximal shortening velocity on activation of the contractile system. Possible mechanism(s) underlying the effect of sarcomere length and Ca_o^{2+}, on velocity of shortening have been investigated in the studies reported in this chapter. The effect of sarcomere length on force development will be presented for comparison. Sarcomere dynamics were investigated in thin trabeculae from Rat heart with laser diffraction techniques, while relations between force and velocity of sarcomere shortening were measured with the use of the 'isovelocity' technique.[1]

It is likely that stretch increases force development predominantly through its effect on sensitivity of the actin-bound troponin to calcium, whereas the velocity of shortening of the unloaded contractile system has been shown to correlate well with the ATPase activity of myosin and therefore probably corresponds to the cycling rate of the cross bridges. In this chapter we have summarized our studies on the effects of interventions that affect either one of the above mechanisms or which affect both. The effects of length, Ca_o^{2+} pH and hypertrophy mediated changes in myosin ATPase enzyme activity on the F–V–SL relation will be reviewed.

Methods

The methods that were used have been described elsewhere.[4] In short, trabeculae were dissected from Rat heart after excision of the heart under ether anesthesia.

The preparation was then mounted between a force transducer and a lever arm. The position of the arm was controlled by a motor. A laser beam was directed through the preparation. The sarcomeres of the preparation acted as a grating causing a diffraction pattern of the laser beam. The central beam was used to observe the muscle via a microscope. A suitable area for the laser diffraction study of sarcomere length could be selected in this way. Areas showing only slight movements during contraction were chosen for measurements of sarcomere lengths. The first order beam was projected onto a photodiode-array. The position of the first order beam measured from the array was used to calculate sarcomere length. Correction was made for scattering of light from the zero order beam. Two different systems were used for the calculations. Their values did not differ significantly from each other. The system was calibrated before each experiment.

The preparations were superfused with a modified Krebs-Henseleit solution containing (in mM):

Na^+ 141.0, K^+ 5.0, Cl^- 127.5, Mg^{2+} 1.2, $H_2PO_4^-$ 2.0, SO_4^{2-} 1.2, HCO_3^- 27, glucose 10.1, Ca^{2+} 0.3 to 4.0; 24–26 C.

To modify pH in the cells solutions were in equilibrium either with 95% O_2 and 5% CO_2 or with 80% O_2 and 20% CO_2. The pH in the first was 7.35 ± 0.02, in the latter 6.68 ± 0.02. Further variations in the gas mixture allowed to change pH over a wider range.

At any SL peak force was measured in the test beat after four twitches at reference length. To measure sarcomere shortening velocity we induced isovelocity releases as previously described.[1,6] Figure 1 shows the release procedure. Muscle length, sarcomere length and force were recorded as a function of time. The preparation was stretched in order to keep sarcomere length constant early during the twitch. The length control system was then switched to load control and the load was varied. The shortening velocity was related to the load.

Another release procedure, used as well, is also illustrated in Fig. 1. Ramps were used to control movements of the lever arm. The first stretch was again used to keep sarcomere length of the observed area constant. A rapid release of controlled amplitude was used to release the preparation to a selected force. This was followed by a release at a controlled velocity to keep the force constant. This method was referred to as the isovelocity release technique. It can be seen in the figure that traces of load-clamp and of the

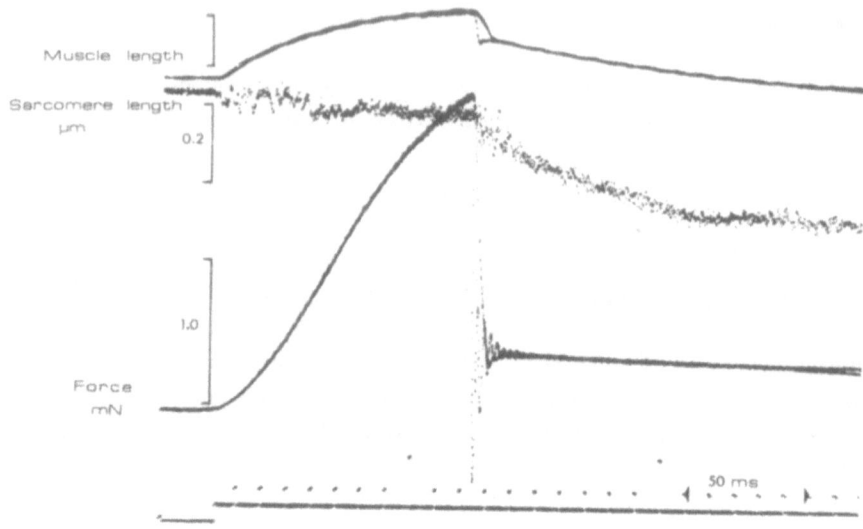

Fig. 1. Contractions of a trabecula at $Ca_o^{2+} = 2.5$ mM. Load clamps and releases at controlled velocity are superimposed. The record shows 15% initial stretch (top trace) of the muscle (length 3.4 mm) needed to keep sarcomere length constant (second trace) at 2.1 μm. Force development (bottom trace) was followed by a release to constant load during which sarcomere shortening occurred. Velocity was measured during the first 50 ms at which load was constant. Alternatively the initial period of contraction at constant SL was followed by a quick release of the muscle to attain the same force. This release was followed by a release at controlled velocity at which the force stayed constant. There releases resulted in identical force records and identical F–V relations (from Daniels et al., J Physiol 355: 367–381).

isovelocity release were virtually superimposable. However, fewer oscillations occurred with the velocity clamp. By means of a least squares statistical approach a rectangular hyperbola, according Hill's equation $(P + a)v = b(P_o - P)$, was fitted on the obtained data. Figure 2 shows the procedure for measurements of the velocity of sarcomere shortening at zero load. Early in the contraction the preparation was stretched in order to keep the sarcomere length of the preparation constant; then ramps were imposed in order to release the preparation to zero load. It is clear from the figure that using ramps with higher velocities did not affect the sarcomere shortening trace. By this procedure it was possible to directly measure V_o.

Results

The force sarcomere length relation

Figure 2 shows the F–SL relation under control conditions and shows the effect of lowering Ca_o^{2+} from 1.5 to 0.3 mM at pH = 7.35.

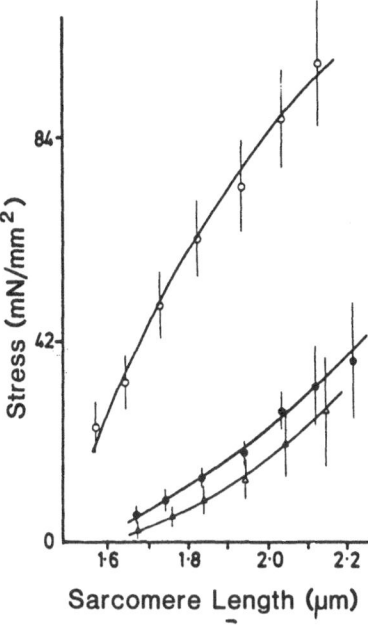

Fig. 2. The relationship between force and sarcomere length at varied Ca^{2+}: 1.5 mM (open circles) and 0.3 mM (open triangles) at pH 7.35. The filled circles indicate the F–SL relation at $Ca_o^{+1} = 1.5$ mM but at pH 6.68. Values of F are indicated ± 1 sem(n = 7). (Redrawn from reference 8.)

Similar results have been obtained with trabeculae from hypertrophied hearts of rat that had been treated with thyroid hormone or in which hypertrophy was induced by hypoxia. This observation suggests that the mechanism responsible for the change of force with change in sarcomere length in normal and hypertrophied muscle is similar. The similarity is consistent with the reported effects of hypertrophy that seems to affect the myosin enzyme system selectively without modifying the troponin dependent Ca^{2+} sensitivity. Lowering Ca^{2+} causes a length dependent decrease of peak twitch force such that the relation which is typically lower toward the ordinate at high Ca_o^{2+} becomes convex toward the abscissa. This well known length dependent effect of Ca_o^{2+} [1,4] is explained (see Chapter 1) by length dependence of the sensitivity of the contractile filament system alone. It can completely be mimicked by the immediate effect of reduction of the pH from 7.35 to 6.68 at $Ca_o^{2+} = 1.5$ mM[8] (see Fig. 2). The change of the F–SL relation shortly after change of pH_i leads to a F–SL relation that is nearly identical to the F–SL relation at normal pH and low Ca_o^{2+}. This observation suggests that the effect of an acute intracellular change of pH, which is not accompanied by a change of calcium release as has been shown by Allen and co-workers[9,10] is to change the sensitivity of the contractile apparatus to

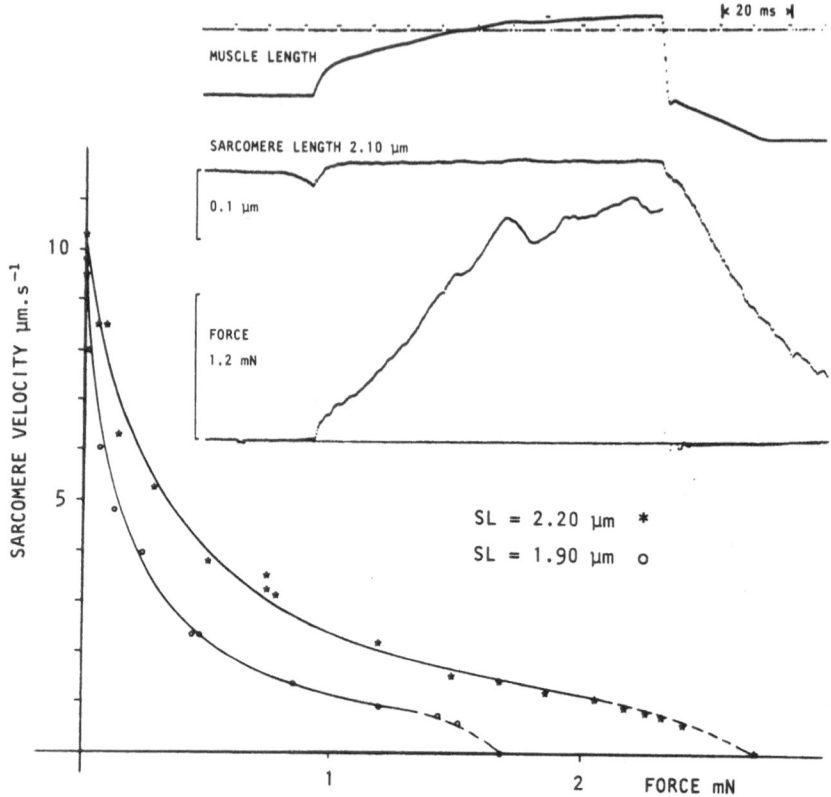

Fig. 3. The inset illustrates the isovelocity release to attain the maximal velocity of shortening. The force velocity relations measured at $Ca_o^{2+} = 2.5$ mM reveal that F_o depends on sarcomere length (asterisks SL = 2.20 μm; circles SL = 1.90 μm) in contrast to V_o which was independent of SL (9.8 μm/s.)

Ca^{2+} in a length-independent manner. This would be consistent with a length independent competition between protons and Ca^{2+} ions for binding to anionic sites of troponin C.

The force–velocity relation and V_o

The force–velocity curve obtained with each of the release techniques is demonstrated in Fig. 3.

In this figure shortening velocity at sarcomere lengths 2.2 and 1.9 μm is related to the load. The results from the two release methods did not differ significantly. There was a slight deviation from a rectangular hyperbola at the highest loads. The same type of deviation has been described for frog

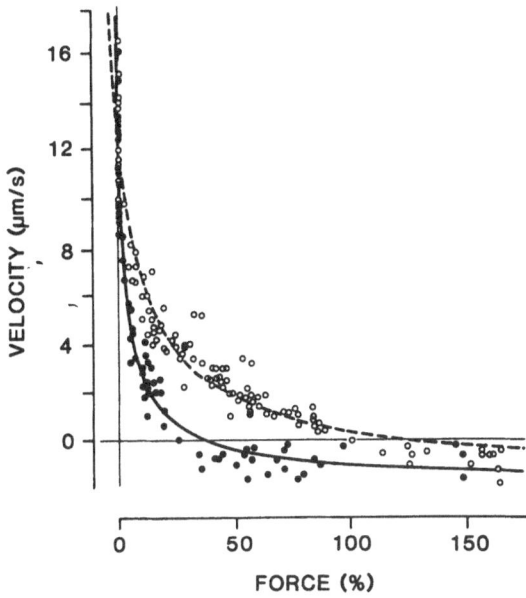

Fig. 4. The relationships between force and velocity at Ca_o^{2+} 1.5 mM; pH *7.35* (open circles) and Ca_o^{2+} 1.5 mM at pH *6.68* (filled circles). Force is expressed as % isometric force at a sarcomere length of 2.00 μm. Note that stretch at a velocity of 1–2 μm/sec cause a fourfold increase in force (filled circles). (From Ricciardi et al., Cardiovascular Research XX, 1986 with permission of the authors).

skeletal muscle[11]. The relation was continuous above P_o for stretches at velocities up to 1 μm/s during which force was maintained at levels up to 400% of F_o (see Fig. 4). It is evident that the enhancement of force by stretch will lend stability to a chain of muscle elements in which force generating capacity may differ such as may occur in ischemic heart disease.

One of the attractive features of the controlled release procedure is that it is possible to study the maximal velocity of sarcomere shortening (V_o) and analyse interventions that affect it directly. It has been shown that the composition of Myosin isoenzymes determines the myosin ATPase activity. Barany has shown that V_o correlates closely with myosin ATPase activity.[12] The prediction that different types of hypertrophy characterized by different isoenzyme expression, are also characterized has been confirmed for shortening velocity in various studies.[13,14] No relation between myofibrillar ATPase activity and velocity of sarcomere shortening is known yet. We adopted therefore three experimental conditions to modify the isoenzyme composition in rat heart. Triiodothyronime induces cardiac hypertrophy with virtually only V_1 isoenzymes. Hypertrophy induced by pressure overload such as results from pulmonary hypertension due to hypoxia is characterized by predominance of V_3 myosin isoenzymes.[15] Trabeculae from the hearts of

Table 1. The comparison of force development and unloaded velocity of shortening in hearts of control animals (C) and after induction of hypertrophy by swimming (S) and triiodothyronime T3). Heartweight (HW) and heartweight to bodyweight (HW/BW) indicate the degree of hypertrophy.

	C	S	T3
HW (mgh)	895 ± 92	1338 ± 164	1355 ± 175
HW/BW	2.88 ± 0.07	4.35 ± 0.38	4.26 ± 0.62
P_o (mN/mm^2)	64.66 ± 7.95	65.25 ± 10.1	64.75 ± 11.92
V_o (μm/sec)	12.25 ± 1.96	13.70 ± 1.58	14.43 ± 1.49
Myosin Ca^{2+} ATPase (μmolP$_i$/min/gww)	17.1 ± 4.4	34.9 ± 4.4	

these animals were compared with those from aged matched controls and muscles form hearts in which hypertrophy was induced by exercise through swimming.[16] The results of the comparison of V_o and myosin ATPase activity are summarized in Table 1. It appeared that indeed V_o and myosin ATPase activity varied concordantly in the different models of hypertrophy, although the quantitative correspondence of V_o and ATPase activity was less strict than expected.[16]

The effect of different calcium concentrations on the force-velocity curve was to decrease both P_o and V_o although to remarkably different extents. Figure 5 demonstrates the relations of V_o and F_o, i.e. velocity and force with the calcium concentration in the perfusate. The calcium concentration was varied between 0.25 and 2.5 mM. P_o at 2.5 mM calcium was taken as 100%. The figure shows that V_o increased with the calcium concentration, but was constant for calcium concentrations above 1.2 mM. V_o was constant when P_o was above about 60% magnitude.

These results would seem to indicate that intracellular calcium determines both the number of active bridges between the filaments and controls the rate of cycling of the bridges.

The time course of increase of V_o and F during the twitch support the notion that both are controlled by Ca_i^{++} although to a different extent. It was observed that V_o rose within 30–40 msec towards a plateau value whereas force continued to increase. Again, V_o was constant for forces above about 50% magnitude. The increase in force and velocity of shortening evidently can be explained by the rise of intracellular calcium during the twitch as a function of time.

The rise of Ca_i^{++} during the twitch would be expected to cause an increase in the number of TnC sites occupied by calcium ions. Could the number of TnC-Ca^{++} complexes then control V_o and F in a differential manner? The number of TnC-Ca^{++} complexes can be modulated at a constant intracellular calcium concentration by varying the sensitivity of TnC to calcium ions.

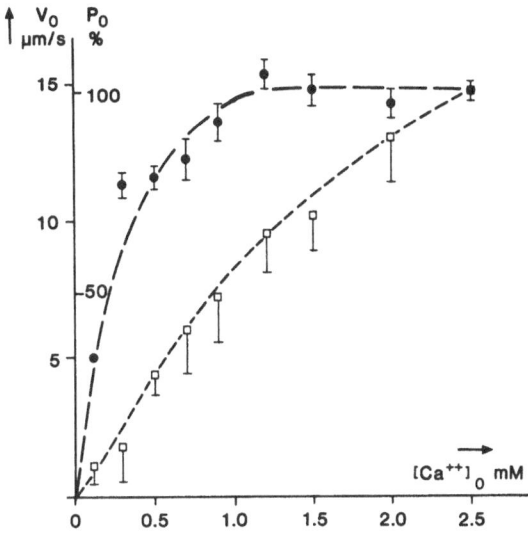

Fig. 5. Shows the relation between unloaded sarcomere shortening V_o (filled circles) and sarcomere isometric twitch force (open squares) at varied $[Ca^{2+}]_o$. V_o was measured at 25 C at SL = 2.00 μm, a length at which internal elastic forces are negligible.

Firstly in Chapter 1 (and above) it has been argued that the sensitivity of TnC can be varied by varying SL.[7] Alternatively it is well known that variation of pH_i will vary the effect of calcium ions by competitive inhibition of binding to TnC. The results of variation of SL and pH provided indeed (indirect) support for the above hypothesis of differential control of V_o and F by the number of TnC-Ca^{++} complexes.

Figure 6 shows that V_o increased with sarcomere length between 1.6 and 1.85 μM. At sarcomere lengths longer than about 1.85–1.90 μm V_o was constant. The regression lines in the figure were calculated for each experiment. The possible contribution of opposing forces of unknown-magnitude at SL's < 1.85 μM evidently warrants caution in the interpretation of this result. Still, it is striking that again, V_o was constant for forces above about 60% maximal force at SL = 2.2 μm.

An alternative way to test the hypothesis that the amount of Ca^{2+} bound to TnC determines V_o is to vary the pH at a constant external calcium concentration and at SL = 2.00 μm. The effect of opposing forces is then avoided. Acidosis (pH 6.68 at Ca_o^{2+} = 1.5 mM) had the same effect on the F–V relation, $(P + a)v = b(P - P_o)$ as lowering Ca_o^{2+} (to 0.3 mM) without a change in pH (see Fig. 4); i.e. the parameter a decreases threefold (from 12.4 to 3.7) whereas the parameter b did not change significantly. Following the decrease of pH twitch force recovered after a transient undershoot in approximately 15 min to maximally 40–45% of control. V_o decreases to 9.5 μm/s

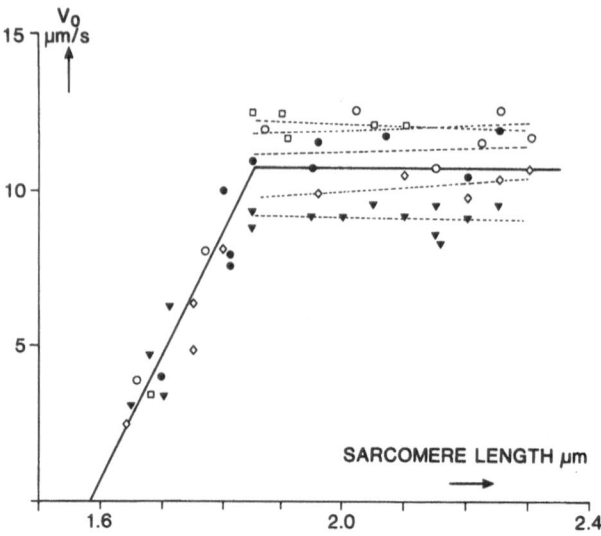

Fig. 6. Shows that at $Ca_o^{2+} = 2.5$ mM V_o is independent of SL between 1.85 μm and 2.3 μm in Rat cardiac muscle at 25 C (Redrawn from reference 1).

both with a decrease of Ca_o^{2+} to 0.3 mM and immediately following a decrease of pH to 6.68 at Ca 1.5 mM. The two interventions led to an equal drop of force. When force recovered during acidosis to approximately 45% of maximal force the velocity of shortening returned to control values (12.5 μm/s).[8]

Discussion

The differential responses of force development and unloaded shortening velocity during the twitch to variation of sarcomere length, or to variation of the Ca^{2+} and H^+ concentrations are consistent with the hypothesis that force development and unloaded velocity of shortening are controlled by different mechanisms. The results, at first glance, seem to indicate that sarcomere shortening velocity is determined directly or indirectly by the intra cellular calcium concentration[1] up to a certain level of intracellular calcium above which shortening velocity is constant. The intracellular calcium concentration and increases transiently following the release of calcium by the sarcoplasmic reticulum that is triggered by the actionpotential.

Shortening velocity if measured at $Ca_o^{2+} = 2.5$ mM also depends on sarcomere length up to SL = 1.9 μm and remains constant at longer sarcomere lengths. This contrasts both force which rises monotonically with SL and calcium release which is independent of SL over the full range of lengths.[1] It is therefore likely that V_o does not simply vary with free Ca^{2+} in the cell but with the amount of Ca^{2+} bound to the contractile systems as reflected by force. The effect of acidosis to lower V_o is consistent with this hypothesis since competition of protons for the binding sites for calcium on TnC would lower the actual amount of bound calcium. This is the more likely because a direct effect of pH on the myosin ATPase rate, and thereby on V_o,[17] only occurs at pH_i levels that are lower than in the studies reported here.[8] A further observation that emerged from these studies is that V_o reaches a maximal value under conditions at which force is approximately 40–60% of maximal force at SL = 2.00 μm and at Ca_o^{2+} = 2.5 mM. This is a surprising finding as one would predict intuitively that cycling of only a few cross-bridges should be sufficient to maintain a maximal velocity of shortening in an unloaded muscle which exhibits a very small frictional force.

The possibility that Ca^{2+} directly influences the myosin ATPase rate in cardiac muscle directly is unlikely. Alternatively, these observations would be consistent with the hypothesis that the myosin ATPase activity depends on the number of available actin sites. One can estimate this number from the developed force, which is attained during the twitch in the intact muscle at Ca_o^{2+} = 1.5–2.5 mM to be approximately 70% of the force at saturating free Ca_i^{2+}.[18] It follows less than 30% of the TnC is occupied and less than 30% of the available actin sites are exposed when F equals 40% of peak twitch force. However, if indeed positive cooperativity between Ca^{2+} binding and force development occurs (cf. Chapter 1) the fraction of TnC bound to Ca^{2+} should be substantially lower when no force is developed as is the case during shortening at maximal velocity of shortening. The conclusion based on aequorin studies that a quick release of cardiac muscle indeed causes dissociation of calcium ions from the contractile filaments supports this hypothesis[19]. The consequence of a quick release during a twitch at the moment that force has attained 40% of our reference value must therefore be substantially less than 30% of all the TnC is bound to Ca^{2+}, and possibly be close to 10% of all TnC. Hence the concentration of exposed action would be in the order of 100 μM. Biochemical evidence[20] has suggested that actomyosin ATPase activity is indeed limited by the action concentration if the action is less than 100 μM.

V_o, therefore, appears to depend on the amount of Ca^{2+} that is bound to the contractile filaments – whether this amount varied as a result of varied Ca_o^{2+}, SL, pH or time of the twitch – under conditions in which only a small fraction of the actin sites is exposed to crossbridges. According to this hypothesis, one would predict that the shortening velocity during the relaxation phase will decrease much more rapidly than isometric force because of the effect of the quick release to zero force to dissociate a substantial amount of Ca^{2+} from TnC. The dissociated Ca^{2+} will largely be taken up by the SR and remaining fraction of TnC bound to Ca^{2+} will be small, resulting in deactivation. Consequently V_o should decrease much more rapidly than isometric force during relaxation. Preliminary experiments confirmed indeed a rapid decrease of V_o.[1,5]

Conclusions

The observations reported here can be phrased in a simple model of actomyosin interactions: Ca^{2+} release by the sarcoplasmic reticulum leads to binding of Ca^{2+} ions to the anionic sites on troponin C. The binding and/or dissociation of calcium is sarcomere length dependent and leads to disinhibition of tropomyosin. As a result, a number of actin molecules becomes available for interaction with myosin crossbridges. Increase of the number of actin sites causes obviously more force development. Force will thus increase with sarcomere length (see Chapter 1) Ca_o^{2+}, free Ca_i^{2+} and pH. The effect of Ca_o^{2+} and pH are similar and suggest that the sensitivity of the filaments to Ca^{2+} varies with pH independent of the length of the sarcomere.

In a similar manner one can envisage the effect of sarcomere length Ca^{2+} and pH on the maximal velocity of shortening if one assumes that the ATP hydrolysis rate is limited in the presence of a low concentration of exposed actin similar to the limited ATPase activity that has been observed in biochemical studies at low actin concentrations ($< 100\ \mu M$)[20].

A prediction that follows rather directly from this hypothesis is that when force decreases with lowering of Ca_o^{2+} the sarcomere length at which the F–SL relation exceeds the level of F, which equals 40% of F at SL = 2.0 μm and at Ca^{2+} = 2.5 mM, should shift to higher SL; therefore, the SL above which V_o becomes independent of SL should shift to a higher value as well. This question has not been studied in Rat yet, but it would explain the length dependence of Vo that has been observed[21] in cardiac muscle of species with a shallower F–Ca_o^{2+} such as cat and ferret.[5]

References

1. Daniels M, Noble MIM, ter Keurs HEDJ and Wohlfart B (1984). Velocity of sarcomere shortening in rat cardiac muscle: relationship to force, sarcomere length, calcium and time. J Physiol 355: 367–381.
2. Forman R, Ford LE and Sonnenblick EH (1972). Effect of muscle length on the force–velocity relationship of tetanized cardiac muscle. Circ Res 31: 195–206.
3. Martyn DA, Rondinone JF and Huntsman LL (1983). Myocardial segment velocity at a low load: time, length, and calcium dependence. Am J Physiol 244: H708–714.
4. ter Keurs HEDJ, Rijnsburger WH and van Heuningen R (1980). Tension development and sarcomere length in rat trabeculae. Circ Res 46: 703–714.

5. ter Keurs HEDJ, Rijnsburger WH and van Heuningen R (1980b). Restoring forces and relaxation of rat cardiac muscle. Eur Heart J 1, suppl A, 67–80.

6. van Heuningen R, Rijnsburger WH and ter Keurs HEDJ (1982). Sarcomere length control in striated muscle. Am J Physiol 242: H411–420.

7. Hibberd MG and Jewell BR (1982). Calcium- and length-dependent force production in rat ventricular muscle. J Physiol 329: 527–540.

8. Ricciardi L, Bucx JJJ and ter Keurs HEDJ (1986). Effects of acidosis on force–sarcomere length and force-velocity relations of rat cardiac muscle. Cardiovasc Res XX(2): 117–123.

9. Allen DG and Kurihara S (1980). Calcium transients in mammalian ventricular muscle. Eur Heart J 1, suppl A, 5–15.

10. Allen DG and Kurihara S (1982). The effects of muscle length on intracellular calcium transients in mammalian cardiac muscle. J Physiol 327: 79–94.

11. Edman KAP, Mulieri LA and Mulieri BS (1976). Non-hyperbolic force–velocity relationship in single muscle fibers. Acta Physiol Scand 98: 143–156.

12. Barany M (1967). ATPase activity of myosin correlated with speed of shortening. J Gen Physiol 50: 197–218.

13. Schwartz K, Lecarpentier Y, Martin J-L, Lompre AM, Mercadier JJ and Swynghedauw B (1981). Myosin isoenzyme distribution correlates with speed of myocardial contraction. J Mol Cell Cardiol 13: 1071–1075.

14. Wikman Cofelt J, Reform H, Hollosi G, Rouleau L, Chuck L and Parmley WW (1982). Comparative force–velocity relation and analysis of myosin of dog atria and ventricles. Am J Physiol 243: H391–H397.

15. Kissling G, Rupp H, Malloy L and Jacob R (1982). Alternations in cardiac oxygen consumption under chronic pressure overload: significance of the isoenzyme pattern of myosin. Bas Res Cardiol 77: 255–269.

16. Ricciardi L, ter Keurs HEDJ, van der Laarse A and Vliegen WM (1986). Variazioni meccaniche e strutturali nel miocardio ipertrofico di ratti allenati al nuoto. Boll Soc It Biol Sper LXII: 89–93.

17. Kentish JC and Nayler WG (1979). The influence of pH on the Ca^{2+}-regulated ATPase of cardiac and white skeletal myofibrils. J Mol Cell Cardiol 11: 611–617.

18. Fabiato A (1981). Myoplasmic free calcium concentration reached during the twitch of an intact isolated cardiac cell and during calcium-induced release of calcium from the sarcoplasmic reticulum of a skinned cardiac cell from the adult rat or rabbit ventricle. J Gen Physiol 78: 457–497.

19. Housmans PR, Lee NKM and Blinks JR (1983). Active shortening retards the decline of the intracellular calcium transient in mammalian heart muscle. Science 221: 159–160.

20. Stein LA, Chock PB and Eisenberg E (1981). Mechanism of actomyosin ATPase. Effect of actin on the ATP hydrolysis step. Proc Natl Acad Sci, USA 78: 1346–1350.

21. Noble MIM (1974). Force-velocity relation at different muscle lengths. In The Physiological Basis of Starling's Law of the Heart, Ciba Foundation Symposium 133–136. Amsterdam: North-Holland, Elsevier Excerpta Medica.

7. Similarity and Dissimilarity Between Muscle Force–Length Relationship and Ventricular Pressure–Volume Relationship

K. SAGAWA, W.C. HUNTER, W.L. MAUGHAN, D. BURKOFF & D. YUE

Department of Biomedical Engineering, School of Engineering, The Johns Hopkins University, Baltimore, Maryland, USA

Abstract

Early studies of the end-systolic pressure–volume relation of the left ventricle showed that it was identical to the isovolumic relationship; this contrasted with the isolated muscle end-systolic force–length relation which fell to the right of the isometric relationship. A discrepancy similar to that of isolated muscle appeared in later studies of the intact heart in which ejection fraction was greater. Further investigation showed that the discrepancy between end-systolic and isovolumic pressure was dependent on (1) the instantaneous rate of ejection, (2) the ejected volume up to the time of end systole and (3) the peak ejection rate of the same beat; the first of these factors predominated. These results are similar to those found in isolated heart muscle and led us to add a pressure dependent dashpot and fixed elastance to our time varying elastance model; there appears to be a shortening induced deactivation factor in addition. The effect of contractility on the shape of the force–length relationship was also found in the end-systolic pressure–volume relation of the left ventricle. Low contractility (extrasystoles) gave curves convex towards the volume axis; high contractility (post-extrasystolic beats, dobutamine) gave curves concave to the volume axis.

Introduction

In the Cardiovascular System Dynamics Society Symposium in 1978, Sagawa[1] addressed the following issues concerning the similarities between the muscle mechanics and ventricular dynamics:

1. Frank[2] demonstrated a strong resemblance that the frog ventricular pressure(P)–volume(V) relationship bears to the force(F)–length(L) relationship of skeletal muscles, with specific reference to the influence of the history of contractile events in the same beat on the end-systolic P–V and F–L relations.

H.E.D.J. ter Keurs and M.I.M. Noble (eds), Starling's Law of the Heart Revisited. ISBN 978-94-010-7084-3

2. Early studies in our laboratory[3] on isolated canine ventricles, however, showed a negligibly small degree of history dependent differences in the end-systolic P–V relationship (ESPVR) between isovolumic contractions and ejecting contractions at varied diastolic volumes. Results from other laboratories also showed little effect of history on the ESPVR.[1] This finding on the canine ventricle appeared, in our first thought, to indicate a marked dissimilarity from the end-systolic F–L relationship (ESFLR) of mammalian heart muscles that had been reported to vary significantly with mode of contraction.[4,5]

3. Later studies,[6] which permitted the ventricle to eject much greater fractions of diastolic volume than in earlier studies, showed that the end-systolic pressures of steady-state beats with ejection fractions greater than 40% were smaller than isovolumic pressures at the identical volumes. This reduction, called end-systolic pressure deficit, reached 20% of the isovolumic pressures as ejection fraction approached 75%.

4. Thus we rediscovered the similarity that Frank found between muscle endsystolic F–L relation and ventricular end-systolic P–V relation because both relations were affected, though not as markedly as he claimed, by the history of preceding contractile events. The diastolic instantaneous P–V relationship showed even a greater effect of systolic history.

In the present paper, we would add to the list of similarity a few recent findings on the ventricular P–V relationship with reference to corresponding studies on heart muscle.

Instantaneous F–L relation vs. P–V relation

Using isolated rabbit papillary muscles, Leach and Brady[7] analyzed the difference in instantaneous muscle force when it is isometrically twitching at a certain length as opposed to when it is shortening at variably controlled speeds around the same length. The shortening muscle force $Fs^{(t)}$ was always smaller than the isometric force $F_{im}(t)$ by an amount linearly proportional to the shortening velocity dl/dt:

$$F_s(t)/F_{im}(t) = 1 + m(dl/dt) + b \qquad (1)$$

The coefficient m increased with the duration (and therefore, extent) of shortening. This indicates that both shortening velocity and extent contribute to the force deficit. The force deficit amounted to 10 to 35% at shortening velocities of 1/2 to 2/3 muscle-length/sec and the shortening extent of 1.7 to 7%.

Leach and Brady[7] consider that the mechanism responsible for the velocity-dependent force deficit must be the same as that underlying the force–velocity relationship, whereas the mechanism responsible for the force deficit

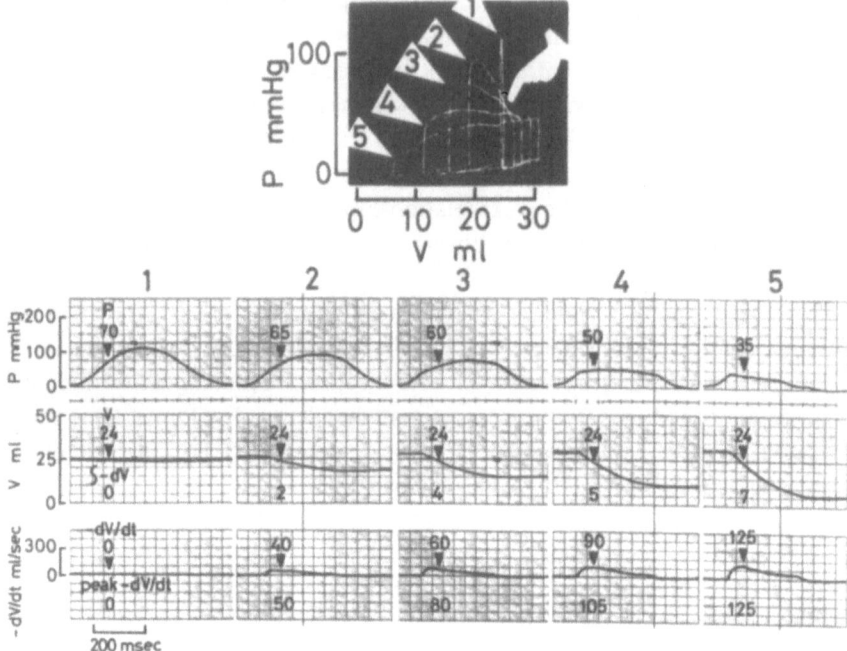

Fig. 1. Top: Oscilloscopic picture of P–V trajectories of 5 contractions of a ventricle. Bottom: Chart recordings of the same 5 contractions. The numbers 1–5 show correspondence. All the contractions are differently preloaded and afterloaded but share the same volume at the same instant of time after the onset of contraction. This can be seen clearly in the bottom panel whereas the difference in ventricular pressure at this time point can be seen clearly in the top panel (pointed out by the indicator). Note in the 3rd channel of the bottom panel that the ventricular outflows (dV/dt) had a similarly physiological wave form, though the peak flow magnitude was markedly varied. Reproduced from Suga et al. (1980) with permission from the American Heart Association, Inc.

dependent on the extent of shortening may be so-called shortening deactivation, i.e., negative manifestation of the length-dependent activation,[8] or of the length-dependent change in Ca^{2+} affininty.[9]

In isolated, blood perfused canine left ventricle, Suga, Sagawa, and Demer[10] determined ventricular pressure P(t) at the same prespecified volume V(t) and at the same time after the onset of contraction with variable ejection rate and ejected volume in the past (Fig. 1). The % reduction of P(t) from $P_{iv}(t)$ was related by the multiple step regression analysis to the instantaneous rate of ejection, dV/dt, the ejected volume up to the time, −dV, and the peak of ejection rate in the past within the same beat, (dV/dt) peak. The analysis gave the following regression equation:

$$P(t)/P_{iv}(t) = 1 - a(-dV/dt) - b(\textstyle\int - dV) - c(-dV/dt)_{peak} \qquad (2)$$

in which t is time after onset of contraction, and a, b, and c are regression coefficients having values of 0.0014, 0.0054 and 0.0007, respectively. When physiological magnitudes of aortic flow, its peak value and ejected volume for various times during ejecting contraction substituted in the equation, the dV/dt term was found to be predominantly important. In view of this new result we modified our old model of ventricular contraction, which consisted of a single time-varying elastance (Fig. 2, left) to the 3-element model shown in the right by the dashpot in parallel and those of the past event by another elastance in series with the time-varying elastance.

We submit that this finding on the ventricular P–V relationship is highly consonant with the finding on the force deficit described above in shortening muscle; the close mechanistic tie between the phenomena observed at the muscle level and at the ventricular level is beyond doubt in our mind.

In the studies described above, the effect of timing of shortening or ejection with respect to the phases of systole was inseparable from the effect of the cumulative amount of ejection because the ejection (or muscle shortening)

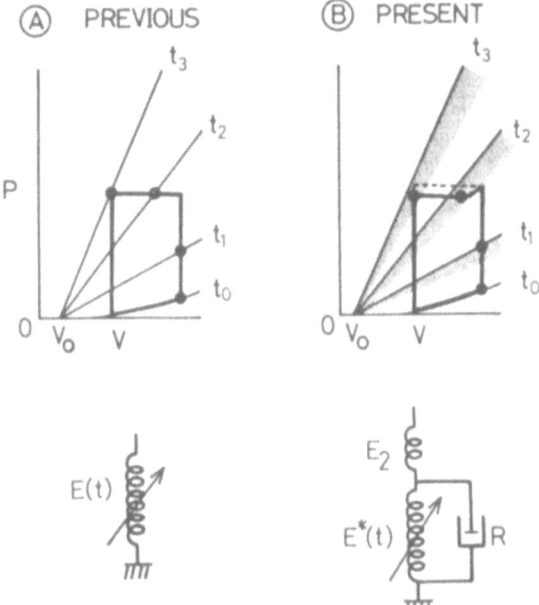

Fig. 2. Illustration of the earlier (A) and recent (B) concept of the instantaneous P–V relationship (top panels) and mechanical analogues (bottom panels). The shaded area beneath the solid lines at t_0, t_1, t_2, and t_3 indicates the reduction of pressure from the isovolumic pressure at the same volume and the same time. Equation 2 describes this pressure reduction. In retrospect, the earlier model (a single time-varying elastance) was conceived from those data with limited ejection fractions (<40%). The $E^*(t)$ in the recent model (bottom panel) indicates $E(t)$ specific for isovolumic condition. Reproduced form Suga et al. (1980) with permission from the American Heart Association, Inc.

went on continuously. Hunter et al[11] could separate the time factor by giving a mild (S-shaped) volume step change to isolated canine ventricles that were otherwise contracting isovolumically and by changing the time at which this volume perturbation V was given at the early, middle or late phase of systole (Fig. 3). The volume step was either positive (infusion) or negative (ejection). The resultant change in ventricular pressure P(t) could be described by the following equation:

$$\Delta P(t)/\Delta V = E(t)B(T) + R(dV/dt)/V - \delta D_T(t). \tag{3}$$

The first term on the right side of the equation represents an elastic property which contributed to P(t) caused by the volume step. It is determined by a product of E(t), an active time-varying elastance, and a modifier, B(T), which depends on the time interval T between the onset of contraction and the instant of V injection; B decreases as T increases, but is constant after the V injection. The second term represents a viscous resistance factor of P which is dependent on the shortening property of heart muscle. The coefficient R appears to be time-varying because it is a linear function of the isovolumic ventricular pressure $P_{iv}(t)$ (Fig. 4, left panel). Its value increases with positive inotropic interventions in proportion to the increase in $P_{iv}(t)$ by the interventions. The last term represents a deactivation component D_t of P which represents a depressive effect of the displacement itself regardless of the direction of V (whether ejection or infusion). The symbol is $+1$ when $V > 0$ and -1 when $V < 0$. D_t is a complex function of time t but its magnitude remains minimal except towards the end of systole. Each of the components of P(t) is illustrated in Fig. 3.

Hunter et al.[11] also consider that the proportional increase of R with P(t) probably reflects the force-velocity relation of the heart muscle. The Hill equation can be arranged in the form of $(F_o - F)/(dl/dt) = F/b + a/b$, in which a and b are the force and velocity constants, respectively. The left side term corresponds to R in Equation 3 and is proportional to F as indicated by the first term on the right hand side of the equation. The finding that R was affected by changes in contractility insofar as P(t) was affected had been reported by another investigator[12] and was reconfirmed by Schroff, Janicki, and Weber et al.[13] The apparent similarity of the ventricular pressure-ejection rate relation muscle force–velocity relation deserves further investigation.

A dissimilarity between muscle internal resistance and ventricular internal resistance is expected to emerge with respect to the influence of preload. Because of the cubic relation of volume to length, a given volume rate of ejection from a larger ventricle will be associated with a slower average shortening velocity of its wall fiber than that of a smaller ventricle ejecting the same volume flow. As a result, that R value calculated at a larger volume will have to be smaller than that for the same ventricle at a smaller volume

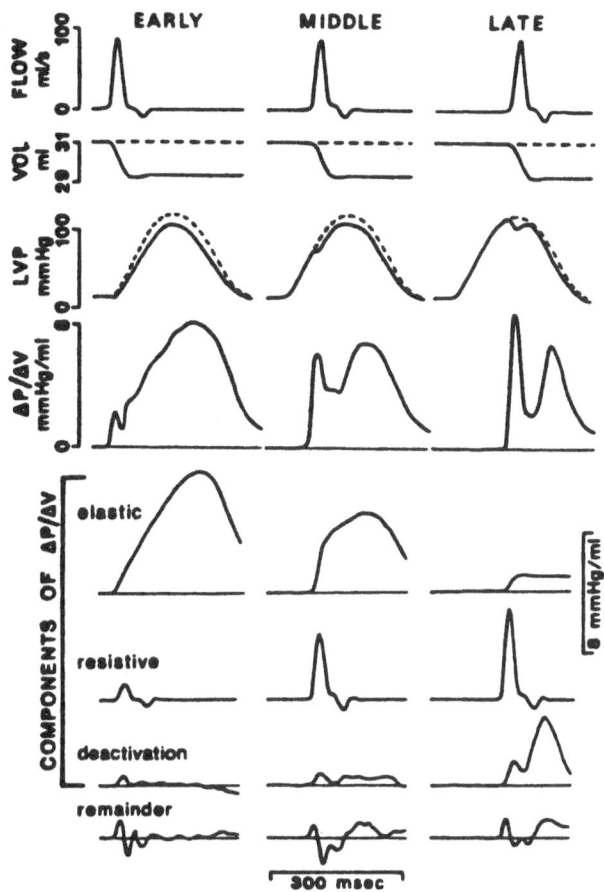

Fig. 3. Volume perturbations given to isovolumically contracting ventricle at early, middle, and late times in systole. Note in the 2nd channel that the volume change is not "instantaneous". In the 3rd channel, the broken curve indicates the isovolumic pressure wave that would have been if there had been no volume change. The difference between this isovolumic pressure and actual pressure with volume perturbation is denoted by P and shown in the 4th channel after normalization by the magnitude of input volume change V. The 5th, 6th and 7th channels show the elastic, resistive, and deactivation component of ventricular pressure response to volume perturbation (P/ V), respectively. These correspond to the three terms on the right of Equation 3. The 8th channel indicates the residual of the response. Note the marked difference in magnitude of each component with time (T in Equation 3) at which the volume perturbation was given. Reproduced from Hunter et al. (1983) with permission from the American Heart Association, Inc.

if R reflects the muscle internal resistance. Hunter et al.[11] found the R value for a ventricle to slightly decrease with increase in its cavity volume (Fig. 4, right panel). This corroborates the above thought. At any rate, the results from Hunter's analysis of internal resistance requires the dashpot in the modified version of Suga and Sagawa's model to be made dependent on pressure.

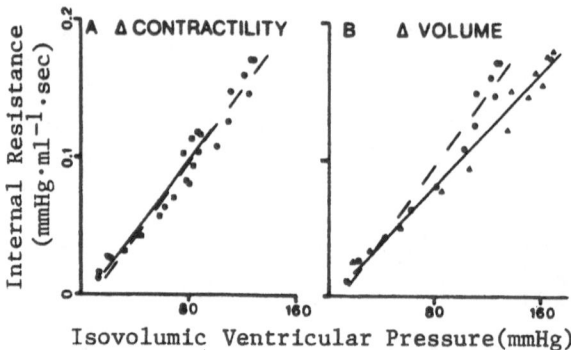

Fig. 4. Plot of internal resistance (R in Equation 3) as a function of instantaneous isovolumetric pressure $P(t)_{iso}$. A: R under control and enhanced contractile states, are both plotted. They are indistinguishable because their relations to $P(t)_{iso}$ are not affected by contractility change. B: the Rs before (broken line) and after (solid line) a considerable change in diastolic ventricular volume. Reproduced from Hunter et al. (1983) with permission from the American Heart Association, Inc.

The deactivation factor DT most probably reflects the marked decoupling effect of sudden length change (regardless of stretch or shortening) on muscle force reported by Bodem and Sonnenblick.[14] The reason for the relatively small magnitude of D_t in Hunter et al.'s study is the relatively slow change of the volume used in their experiment compared with those step length changes in muscle experiments.[14] B(T) has not yet been recognized in muscle studies. It is difficult to represent it by a component of the standard mechanical analog of physical systems.

Elzinga and Westerhof[15] also tested the single elastance model of ventricular contraction on the basis of muscle mechanics. They made cat trabecula undergo variably afterloaded contractions, all from an identical initial length, so that the F(t) and L(t) could be converted into P(t) and V(t) variables via a cylindrical model of the ventricular geometry and the time course of the converted P(t) and V(t) would be as shown in the top panel of Fig. 5. They then analyzed isochronous sets of P(t) – V(t) relationships from these P(t) – V(t) data to see if E(t) lines were similar to those reported by Suga and Sagawa.[3] An example of their results is shown in the bottom panel of Fig. 5 which indicates that E(t) lines shift in an almost parallel fashion from the right lower corner towards the left upper corner rather than changing their slope like a fan around a nearly constant V_o. Because of this difference between the E(t) projected from muscle contraction and the E(t) reduced from ventricle, Elzinga and Westerhof concluded that the behavior of the canine ventricle as a single time-varying elastance might be related to the complex organization of the cardiac muscle fibers in the wall rather than the fundamental muscle property.

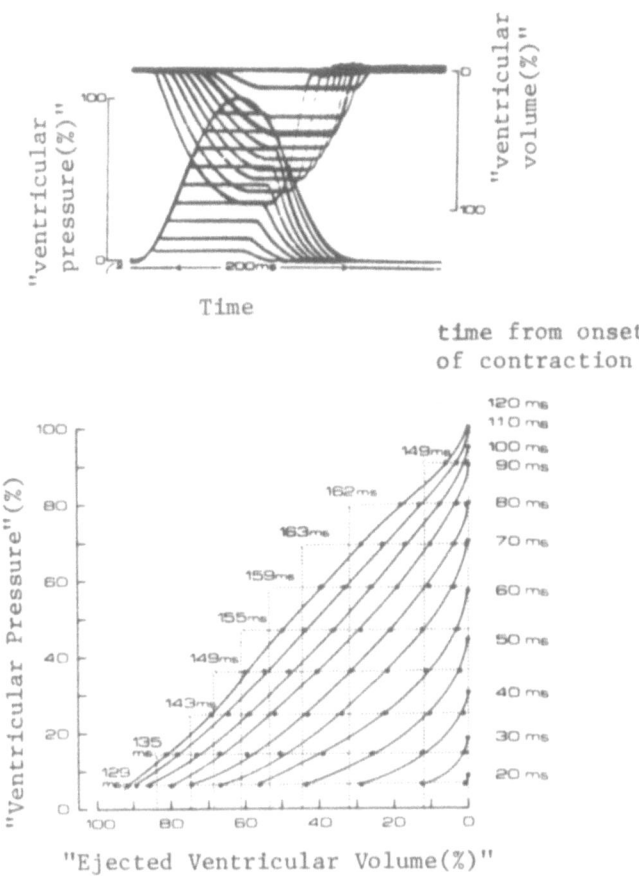

Fig. 5. Elzinga and Westerhof's experiment to estimate ventricular "pressure–volume" relationship from excised cat papillary muscle contraction. The "pressure" and "volume" were computed on-line from muscle force and length using a cylinder model of ventricular geometry coupling the "ventricle" with variable aortic input impedance so that the pressures and volumes shown in the top panel would result. The bottom panel shows the time-varying "volume elastance" lines E(t) deduced form the muscle contractions. Note its similarity to those E(t) line in the bottom panel of Fig. 6 and dissimilarity to those E(t) in the top panel. Reproduced form Elzinga and Westerhof (1981) with the permission of the American Heart Association, Inc.

The dissimilarity in E(t) revealed by Elzinga and Westerhof, however, could have derived from the difference in loading conditions between their experiment and Suga and Sugawa's study.[3] In the latter, the ventricular afterload resistance was kept constant while the preloaded volume was varied extensively. We[16] recently addressed this issue specifically by comparing two E(t)s: one E(t) from ventricular contractions afterloaded with constant afterload and varied preload and the other from contractions with constant preload and varied afterload. As illustrated by the examples in the left and right panels of Fig. 6, the former type loading produced E(t)s changing like

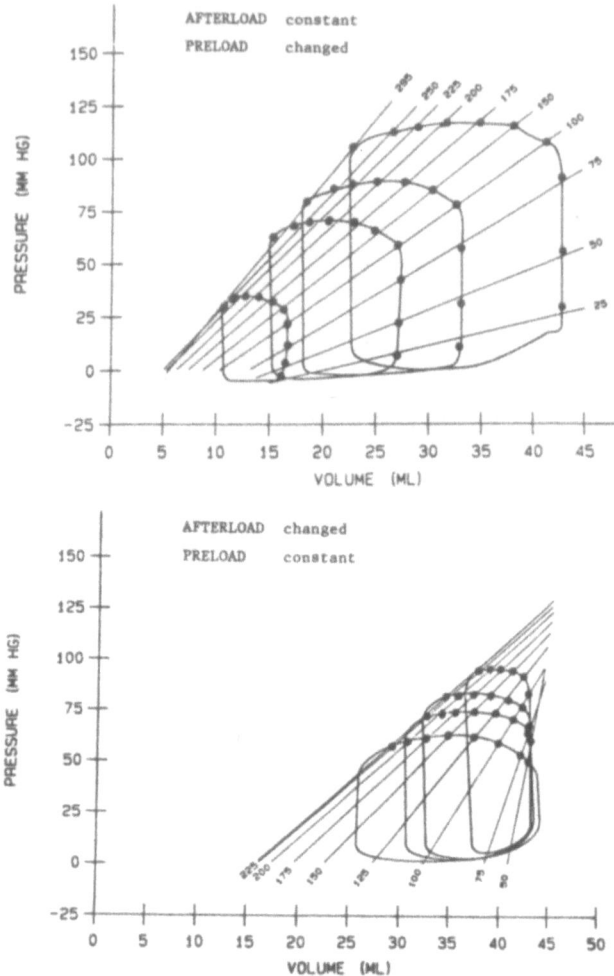

Fig. 6. Effect of loading conditions on instantaneous volume elastance E(t). Top: arterial impedence afterloaded on an isolated ventricle was kept constant while preloaded end-diastolic volume
was varied at 4 values. Bottom: resistance afterloaded on an isolated ventricle was varied at 4
values while preloaded end-diastolic volume was kept constant. Note the similarity of the chance
in E(t) line with time in the top panel to that shown schematically in Fig. 2, but the dissimilarity
to that shown in Fig. 5. Reproduced from Maughan et al. (1985) with the permission from the
Federation of American Society for Experimental Biology.

a fan whereas the latter type loading produced E(t)s shifting in parallel as
predicted from variably afterloaded muscle contractions by Elzinga and
Westerhof. Therefore, we conclude that the architectural complexity of the
ventricle has little to do with the seeming dissimilarity between muscle E(t)
and ventricular E(t). Rather the internal (effective) resistance R seems to be
responsible for the disparate E(t)s observed with different combinations of
preload and afterload conditions, whether in muscle or in the ventricle.

End-systolic F–L and P–V relationships

Effect of loading conditions

We[6] defined end of ventricular systole as the peak of its contractile activity. For isovolumic contraction, end systole thus defined is the time of peak pressure. For ejecting contraction, it is not necessarily the end of ejection but the time at which a ratio of ventricular pressure to volume, defined as $E(t) = P(t)/[V(t - V_o(t)]$ becomes maximum (t_3 in Fig. 2). $V_o(t)$ in this equation is determined as the volume axis intercept of the regression lines drawn for isochronous sets of $P(t$–$V(t)$ data points. The slope of the end systolic $E(t)$ line is termed E_{max}. In the left ventricle, ejection ends under physiological conditions at almost the same time as end systole defined above. When the afterloaded aortic impedance is very low, as is physiologically the case with the right ventricle, the end of ejection occurs much later than end systole.[6]

Presented schematically in Fig. 7 are the results of our study in which computer simulated aortic impedance was afterloaded on isolated ventricles and the effect of changing the preload and afterload in different combinations on ventricular ESPVR were studied.[17] When the preload volume was changed while keeping the afterload resistance at a constant physiological level, the

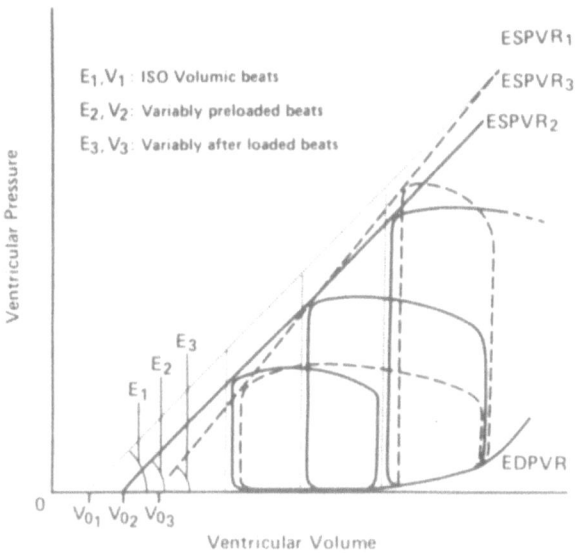

Fig. 7. Schematic presentation of three end-systolic pressure–volume relationship lines (ES-PVR$_{1,2}$ and $_3$) in the P–V diagram. ESPVR$_1$ is obtained from isovolumic contractions, ESPVR$_2$ from contractions against a constant impedance afterload but from different end-diastolic volumes, and ESPVR$_3$ from contractions against drastically different afterload impedances but from a constant end-diastolic volume.

ESPVR shifted in a parallel fashion to the right of the isovolumic ESPVR. Thus the slope remains the same. When the preload volume was kept at a constant volume and the afterload resistance is changed tremendously from infinity (isovolumic condition) to a physiological value, and then to a subphysiologically low value, the ESPVR is altered such that both the slope and volume axis intercept increase. The slope of ESPVR lines is denoted by E_{es}, rather than E_{max}, because the ESPVR here is obtained by drawing a regression line for the upper left corners of the P–V loops, instead of determining multiple E(t) lines and finding the E(t) with a maximal slope.

These effects of afterload resistance can be interpreted as a result of deactivation effects of ejection, $\int - dv$ and $(-dV/dt)$ peak in Equation 2 or $D_t(t)$ in Equation 3. Because there may be a small flow at end systole when resistance is normal or a considerable flow when resistance is subphysiological, the internal resistance of muscle and of the ventricle (represented by m in Equation 1 and a in Equation 2 or R in Equation 3, respectively) will have a more or less depressor effect on end-systolic pressure.

All of the data reported on the end-systolic force–length relationship (ESFLR) of muscle were obtained by making muscle contract isometrically at various lengths and then under a series of isotonic afterload tensions from an identical preload length.[4,5] The ESFLR obtained from afterloaded contractions was found to shift from the isometric ESFLR just as the ventricular $ESPVR_3$ shifts from the $ESPVR_1$ in Fig. 7 when afterloaded arterial resistance was altered from infinity to smaller values. Muscle data are missing as to how ESFLR shifts when the afterload impedance for muscle contraction is maintained and the preload length is changed.

Effect of contractility

One of the evidences presented for the concept of length-dependent activation of heart muscle[18] is that inotropic interventions alter the shape of the relationship between dT/dt (T = muscle tension) and length such that the curves obtained with different contractility cannot be superimposed on each other even after normalization for their maximum dT/dt's at an identical length. Shown in the left panel of Fig. 8 is an example of such an effect of inotropic intervention on isometrically contracting rat trabecular force–sarcomere length relationship reported by ter Keurs et al.[19] It indicates that the quasi-linear relationship observed in the control condition was converted into a curvilinear relationship, with a steeper slope in the small length range and shallower slope in the large length range, as a result of increasing the bath calcium concentration from 0.5 mM to 2.5 mM.

Very similar changes in the shape of isovolumically contracting ventricular ESPVR were observed in our laboratory. Isolated canine ventricles were paced at an interval of 600 msec and their contractility was changed once in a while by injecting pairs of extrasystolic and post-extrasystolic stimuli at test intervals TI_1 and TI_2 (with $TI_1 + TI_2 = 1200$ msec). As shown in the right panel of Fig. 8, the ESPVRs derived from the extrasystolic beats were convex towards the volume axis, the convexity being greater for weaker contractions when TI_1 was shorter. In contrast, the ESPVRs derived from the postextrasystolic beats were concave towards the volume axis and the concavity was greater for stronger contractions at longer TI_2. In another set of preliminary experiments with dobutamine, we observed the similar effect of enhanced contractility on the shape of the ESPVR. Thus the manner in which these inotropic interventions alter the curvilinearity of the ESFLR of muscle and the ESPVR of ventricle bear an obvious resemblance, and it is difficult to think that the resemblance is merely fortuitous.

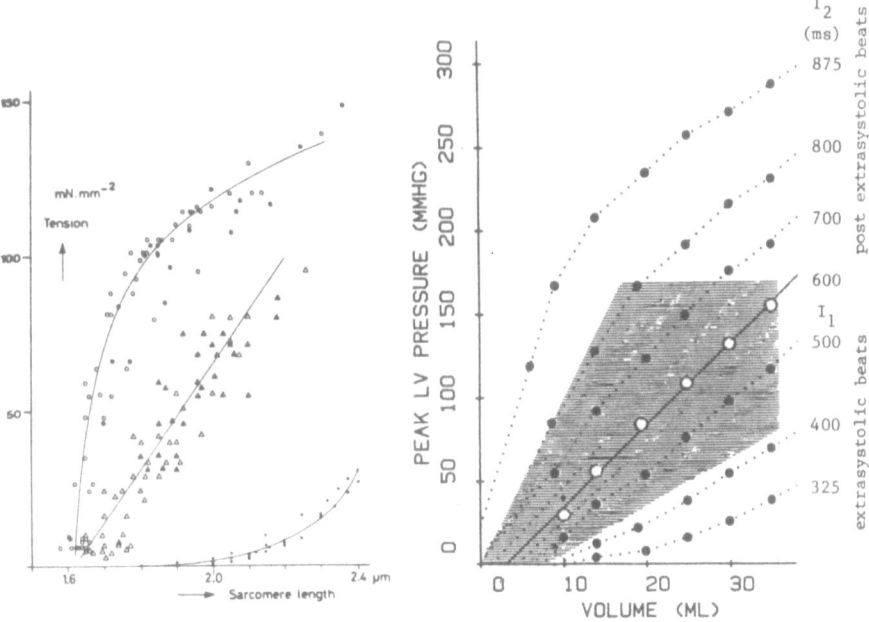

Fig. 8. Influence of contractility on muscle tension–sarcomere length relationship and on ventricular pressure–volume relationship. Left: rat trabecula under control condition (triangles) and augmented contractility with increase in bath $[Ca^{2+}]$ (circles). Reproduced from ter Keurs et al. (1980) with the permission of the American Heart Association, Inc. Right: Canine left ventricle contracting isovolumically under steady control state (open circle) and altered contractile state by sudden change in stimulation interval. Extrasystolic beats with shorter intervals (I_1) than the steady control interval (600 ms) produced those peak)systolic pressure–volume relation curve which are concave upwards, whereas postextrasystolic beats with longer intervals (I_2) produced those peak)systolic pressure–volume relation curve which are convex upwards. Note the similarly curvilinearizing influence of altered contractility on the muscle and ventricular curves.

Incidentally, note that the portions of the ESPVRs falling in the shaded area are approximately rectilinear and that this area is the range of end-systolic pressure and volume with which our past studies have dealt. Therefore, the curvilinear ESPVRs over such an extensive pressure–volume range as shown in Fig. 8 in no way contradicts the thesis we have put forth that acute inotropic interventions significantly increase[3] or decrease[20] the slope of ESPVR without significantly changing its linearity or the volume axis intercept. Nevertheless, we must admit that our concept of the ESPVR as being independent of the preload is a limited one against the wider perspective available now.

Conclusion

We presented several recently acquired evidences for a concept that the ventricular pressure–volume relationship parallels, but is not the same as, the muscle force–length relationship. The evidence includes the similar deactivation effect that reduction of afterload resistance to shortening or ejection exerts on the instantaneous F–L relation and the instantaneous P–V relation, and the similar manner in which inotropic interventions modify the end systolic F–L relation and end-systolic P–V relation. It is obvious that ventricular cavity pressure and cavity volume are related to a certain muscle force and muscle length integrated in a complex way to represent the regional quantitative diversities in these variables. The knowledge of one of the two relationships cannot totally replace the other; rather they complement each other to enrich our understanding of the basic common mechanisms and the different peculiarities for muscle and the ventricular chamber.

References

1. Sagawa K (1978). The ventricular pressure–volume diagram revisited. (Brief Review) Circ Res 43: 677–687.
2. Frank O (1985). Zer Dynamik des Herzmuskels. Z Biol 32: 483–526.
3. Suga H and Sagawa K (1974). Instantaneous pressure–volume relationships and their ratio in the excised, supported canine left ventricle. Circ Res 35: 117–126.
4. Brady AJ (1967). Length–tension relation in cardiac muscle. Am Zoologist 7: 603–610.
5. Taylor RR (1970). Active length–tension relations compared in isometric, afterload and isotonic contractions of cat papillary muscle. Circ Res 26: 279–288.
6. Suga H, Kitabatake A and Sagawa K (1979) End–systolic pressure determines stroke volume from fixed end-diastolic volume in canine left ventricle under constant contractile state. Circ Res 44: 238–249.
7. Leach JK, Brady AJ, Skipper BJ and Millis DL (1980). Effect of active shortening on tension development of rabbit papillary muscle. Am J Physiol 238: H8–H13.
8. Jewell BR (1977). A reexamination of the influence of muscle length on myocardial performance (Brief Review) Circ Res 40: 221–230.

9. Hibberd MG and Jewell BR (1982). Calcium and length-dependent force production in rat ventricular muscle. Physiol (Lond) 329: 527–540.

10. Suga H, Sagawa K and Demer L (1980). Determinants of instantaneous pressure canine left ventricle. Time and volume specification. Circ Res 46: 256–263.

11. Hunter WC, Janicki JS, Weber KT and Noordergraf A (1983). Systolic mechanical properties of the left ventricle: Effects of volume and contractile state. Circ Res 52: 319–327.

12. Templeton GH and Nardizzi LR (1974). Elastic and viscous stiffness of the canine left ventricle. J Appl Physiol 36: 123–127.

13. Shroff SG, Janicki JS and Weber KT (1983). Left ventricular systolic dynamics in terms of its chamber mechanical properties. Am J Physiol 245: H110–H124.

14. Bodem R and Sonnenblick EH (1974). Deactivation of contraction by quick release in the isolated papillary muscle of the cat. Effects of lever damping, caffeine, and tetanization. Circ Res 34: 214–225.

15. Elzinga G and Westerhof N (1981). "Pressure–volume" relations in isolated cat trabecula. Circ Res 49: 388–394.

16. Maughan WL, Sunagawa K, Hunter WC and Sagawa K (1985). Instantaneous but not end–systolic pressure–volume relationship (ESPVR) depends on afterload. Feder Proc 44: 1017.

17. Maughan WL, Sunagawa K and Sagawa K (1984). Effects of arterial input impedance on mean ventricular pressure–flow relation. Am J Physiol 247(16): H978–H983.

18. Lakatta EG and Jewell BR (1977). Length-dependent activation: its effect on the length–tension relation in cat ventricular muscle. Circ Res 40: 251–256.

19. ter Keurs HEDJ, Rijnsburger WH, van Heuningen R and Nagelsmit MJ (1980). Tension development and sarcomere length in rat cardiac trabeculae. Circ Res 46: 703–714.

20. Sunagawa K, Maughan WL, Friesinger GC, Guzman P, Chang M and Sagawa K (1982). Effect of coronary arterial pressure on left ventricular end-systolic pressure–volume relation of isolated canine heart. Circ Res 50: 727–734.

8. The Importance of the Geometry of the Heart to the Pump

T. ARTS,[1] & R.S. RENEMAN[2]

Departments of [1]Biophysics and [2]Physiology, University of Limburg, Maastricht, The Netherlands

Abstract

There is evidence to support the possibility that in the intact heart muscle fibre stress and extent of shortening are homogeneous. If this is assumed to be true, a model of the left ventricle can be constructed where these properties are achieved by appropriate orientation of fibres and torsional movement of the ventricle as a whole. The original cylindrical model was developed into one which was independent of ventricular shape. The equation:

$$P_{lv} = S_f/3 \ \ln (1 + V_w/V_{iv})$$

(where P_{lv} = left ventricular pressure, S_f = fibre stress, V_w = left ventricular wall volume and V_{iv} = left ventricular cavity volume) gives the relationship of muscle force to ventricular pressure. The equation:

$$L_s/L_{So} = [(1 + x)^{1 + x}/x^x]^{1/3}$$

(where $x = V_{lv}/V_w$, L_s = sarcomere length and L_{so} = extrapolated sarcomere length at zero cavity volume) gives the relationship of sarcomere length to ventricular cavity and wall size. The model is equally applicable to mice and elephants and gives realistic ventricular haemodynamic and muscle mechanical values. It can also accommodate the right ventricle, valves, chordae tendinae and papillary muscles.

Introduction

The geometry of the heart plays a major role in the transfer of mechanical energy from the microscopic level of the sarcomeres to the macroscopic level of the left ventricular cavity, where it is used for cardiac pump function. Investigation of this transfer mechanism requires a quantitative description of

H.E.D.J. ter Keurs and M.I.M. Noble (eds), Starling's Law of the Heart Revisited. ISBN 978-94-010-7084-3
© 1988, Kluwer Academic Publishers, Dordrecht

cardiac mechanics in general. At the microscopic level the most relevant parameters are regional values of muscle fiber stress and sarcomere length. At the macroscopic level of the left ventricular cavity, relevant parameters are cavity pressure and volume, aortic and mitral volume flow, and forces within cardiac structures such as the mitral valve, chordae tendinae and papillary muscles. Experimental investigation of the parameters at the macroscopic, hemodynamic level is possible with the use of more or less standard techniques such as pressure and flow measuring devices. However, in the beating heart, direct measurement of mechanical parameters at the microscopic level is complicated. For instance, accurate measurement of local muscle fiber stress is practically impossible. Therefore, instead of experimental investigations, a variety of mathematical models of left ventricular mechanics are in use to study the complex relation between cardiac muscle fiber mechanics and left ventricular pump function.

Generally, the strategy to design a mathematical model of left ventricular mechanics begins with interpretation of a number of physiological findings, obtained in experiments. These findings are combined to a more general idea, which is described in mathematical terms. As a result, the designed model describes the physiological situation most accurately in the vicinity of the physiological conditions, which were the basis of the model. Thus, such models focus on an accurate representation of certain aspects like left ventricular geometry,[1,2,3] matching of observed fiber orientation[4,5,6] transmural differences in mechanical loading[7,8,9] or contractile behavior of the cardiac muscle.[10] In designing models of left ventricular mechanics a major step forward to a more physiological description was made by considering anisotropy of the muscle fiber structure of the heart in combination with the introduction of torsional deformation of the wall of the left ventricle.[11,12,13] Despite the fact that less attention was paid to the geometry of the left ventricle, good agreement was found between model prediction and animal experiments a far as the characteristics of cardiac deformation are concerned.

The model of left ventricular mechanics, as described by Arts et al.,[11,12] appeared to have the striking property that during systole the transmural distribution of muscle fiber stress was quite homogeneous and nearly independent of the state of left ventricular filling. The transmural distribution of fiber stress could be made even more homogeneous by careful adjustment of the transmural course of muscle fiber orientation. This finding gave rise to a new approach in understanding the characteristics of left ventricular mechanics, in which a hypothesis on some ideal, optimal characteristic of the heart is introduced as a basis of cardiac mechanics. When starting from single physiological observations of the real heart, generally it is difficult to obtain an overview of the most significant characteristics. However, when an introduced hypothesis appears to be successful in explaining a wide variety of characteristics, a number of general rules for the design of the cardiac structure may be obtained.

Hypothesis on homogeneous distribution of muscle fiber stress

In the present study, the hypothesis is introduced that muscle fiber stress is homogeneously distributed over all structures of the normal, non-ischemic cardiac ventricles. Furthermore, the mechanical properties of cardiac muscle are assumed to be the same everywhere in the heart. The hypothesis is plausible for a number of reasons. Firstly, studies on the transmural distribution of coronary perfusion, using radioactively labeled microspheres as flow tracer, reveal a quite homogeneous distribution of coronary perfusion within the wall of the left ventricle. Generally the inhomogeneities are less than $\pm 10\%$,[14,15] and appear to diminish with exercise.[16] Secondly, when left ventricular pressure is higher than normal, the left ventricle tends to hypertrophy, resulting in a reduction of muscle fiber stress in the wall to more normal values. Thus, inherently, cardiac muscle tends to keep mechanical load per unit of tissue volume constant. Thirdly, study of the anatomical structure of the muscle fibers in the vicinity of the base and of the apex of the left ventricle reveal that the subendocardial muscle fibers are continuous with the subepicardial ones by crossing over the mid myocardial layers.[18] Thus, muscle fiber stress in the subendocardial and subepicardial layers is likely to be the same. Finally, the local radius of curvature of the wall of the left ventricle appears to be proportional with local wall thickness, as can be observed in long axis cross-sections of the left ventricle, by applying two-dimensional echocardiography. Application of Laplace's law, stating wall tension to be proportional to the radius of curvature, suggests proportionality of wall tension with wall thickness. This finding is also in agreement with constant fiber stress at the various sites in the cardiac wall.

As already mentioned above, mathematical construction of a structure simulating the left ventricle with homogeneous distribution of fiber stress in the wall, appears to be possible. The simplest structure with this property is a cylinder with appropriate transmural course of fiber orientation. Due to cylinder symmetry, instantaneous local mechanical loading in the wall can be described to depend on one single spatial variable: the radial coordinate. Thus, in this case the problem can be reduced to a one dimensional mathematical description. Description of the left ventricular cavity by a sphere is more complicated, because definition of fiber orientation requires definition of an equatorial direction as a reference. As a direct consequence of introducing an equator, the spherical symmetry of the mathematical description is violated. The local mechanical load then depends on two spatial variables: the radial coordinate and the distance to the equator. The problem becomes two-dimensional and is essentially not much simpler than an ellipsoidal geometry of the left ventricle. Because of the simpler mathematical description, the cylindrical geometry is preferred over the spherical geometry in the present study.

Mathematical model of left ventricular mechanics

The design of the mathematical model of left ventricular mechanics has been described earlier,[11,12] and its properties are briefly recapitulated below. The heart is simplified to a left ventricle with a cylindrical geometry (Fig. 1). Cardiac muscle is highly anisotropic and is simplified to a fibrous structure embedded in a soft incompressible material. Fiber orientation in the wall of the right ventricle and septum are considered to be different from the orientation in the free wall of the ventricle. The base of the left ventricle is a thin flexible sheet, containing the aortic and mitral valves. The tips of the flexible mitral valve leaflets are attached to the papillary muscles by the chordae tendineae. The latter muscles are attached to the bottom of the cylinder. Circumferential stresses in the wall of the cylinder generate left ventricular pressure in accordance with Laplace's law. In a cross-section of the cylinder perpendicular to the axis, expelling axial forces due to cavity pressure are in equilibrium with axial stresses in the wall. Shear stresses in the latter cross-section act circumferentially and result in an equilibrium of torques around the cylinder axis. Thus the cylinder is allowed to twist, simulating rotation of the apex with respect to the base around the long axis of the left ventricle. The pumping left ventricle is loaded with a realistic aortic input impedance.

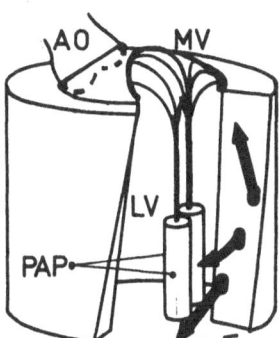

Fig. 1. In a mathematical model of left ventricular mechanics, this ventricle (LV) is represented by a cylinder. The arrows denote muscle fiber orientation. The tips of the mitral valve (MV) leaflets are attached to the papillary muscles (PAP), which in turn are connected to the bottom of the cylinder.

Fig. 2 shows the result of a simulation of a canine cardiac cycle of 600 ms duration. The time course of left ventricular pressure, aortic pressure and aortic volume flow appear to be quite realistic. Mitral backflow occurring during the isovolumic contraction phase is associated with bulging of the mitral valve leaflets towards the left atrium. In the *in vivo* situation this phenomenon is found to occur in a similar way.[19,20] However, ventricular

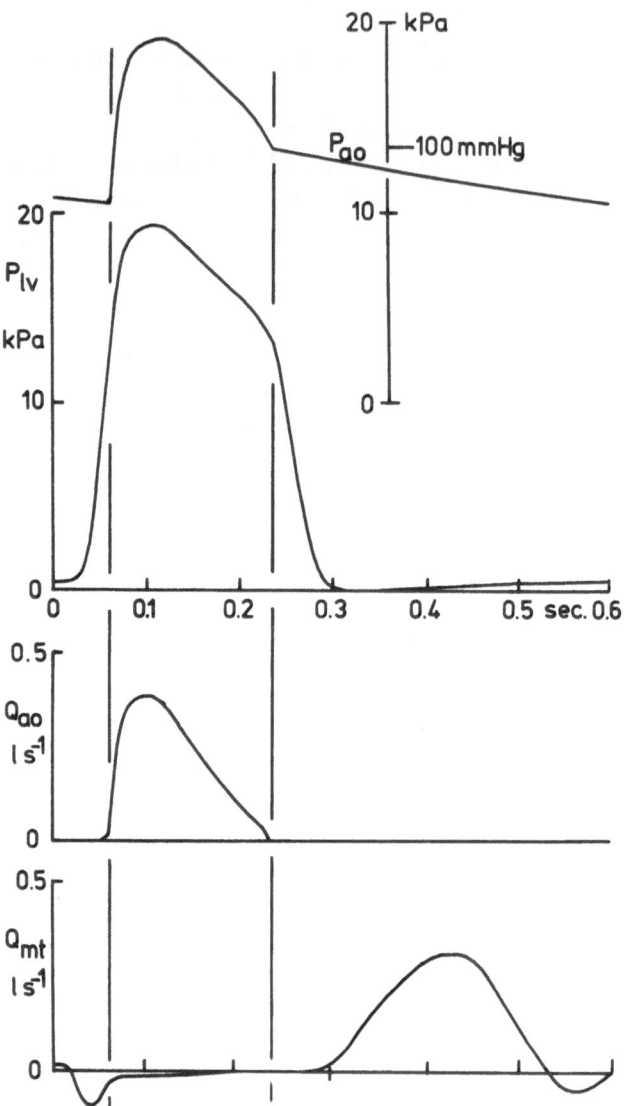

Fig. 2. Simulation of hemodynamical parameters during a normal cardiac cycle. The vertical lines indicate beginning and end of the ejection phase. P_{lv} = left ventricular pressure, P_{ao} = aortic pressure, Q_{ao} = aortic volume flow, Q_{mt} = mitral volume flow. Note the mitral backflow at the beginning of systole.

filling seems to be too slow, which might be due to absence of restoring forces of cardiac muscle in the simultation.

Fig. 3 shows calculated sarcomere length and muscle fiber stress in the various parts of the cardiac muscle as a function of time. During systole sarcomere length as well as fiber stress are approximately the same within the various layers of the ventricular wall as well as the papillary muscles, indicating the possibility to design a structure enclosing a cavity and having the property of homogeneous fiber stress everywhere. Thus our hypothesis is translated into a mathematical model of left ventricular mechanics, which obeys physical laws of equilibria of forces.

Fig. 4 shows calculated loops of left ventricular pressure as a function of left ventricular volume for 3 different end-diastolic volume conditions. Shape and changes in shape of these loops as a consequence of different hemodynamic loading conditions are similar to experimental results reported by Suga et al.[21]

One of the tests on validity of the model is based on comparison of systolic wall deformation, as calculated and as measured directly in physiological experiments. According to the calculations, twisting of the left ventricle around its long axis occurs simultaneously with circumferential shortening. The amount of torsion is quantified by an angle, being the gradient of the

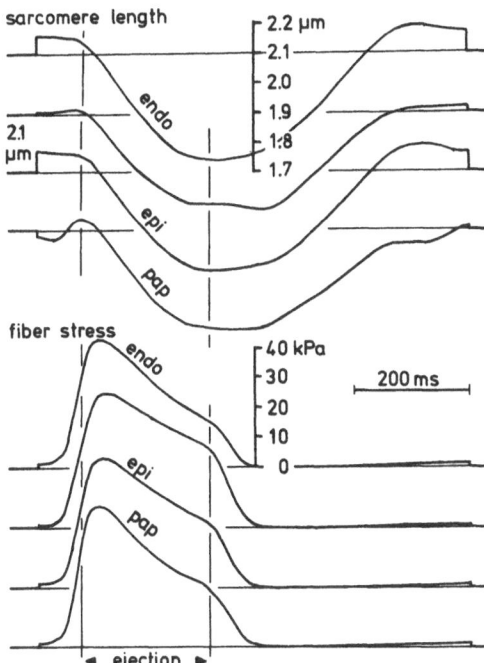

Fig. 3. Simulation of sarcomere length and muscle fiber stress during the same cardiac cycle as presented in Fig. 2. The level at the beginning and ending of each tracing is a calibration level.

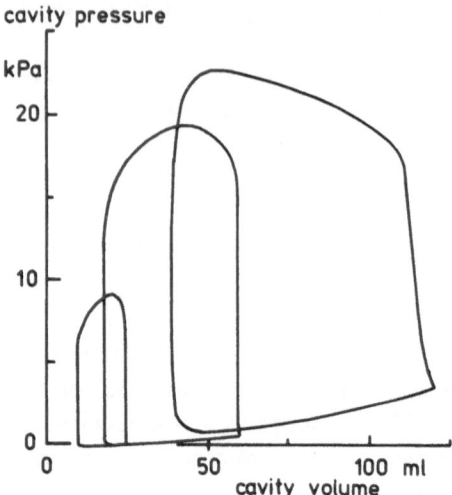

Fig. 4. Pressure–volume plots of 3 simulated heart beats starting at different levels of end-diastolic left ventricular volume (25, 60 = control, and 120 ml).

angle of rotation of the short axis cross-section along the long axis of the left ventricle, multiplied by the outer circumference of the left ventricular wall. Calculation showed that, nearly independent of preload, afterload and contractility, the ratio of circumferential shortening to the torsion angle should be in the narrow range of 2.4 to 2.6. In 9 experiments on closed chest dogs, using two-dimensional echocardiography, this ratio (2.31 ± 0.23; mean $\pm$ sd) was found to be in good agreement with the calculated value.[22] Interestingly, the latter ratio is dimensionless indicating its validity for the hearts of all species, independent of their size; in other words the ratio holds for mice as well as elephants.

Characteristics related to homogeneity of fiber stress

Introduction

In the present study the mathematical model of the mechanics of the left ventricle is used as a tool to obtain a more general understanding of geometric features in relation to conversion of muscle fiber work to left ventricular pumping work. Special attention is paid to: a) the transmural course of fiber orientation in relation to the transmural distribution of mechanical work done by muscle fibers, b) the relation between left ventricular pressure and volume on the one hand, and muscle fiber stress and sarcomere length on the other, c) the relation between the ratio of left and right ventricular weight and the work to be done by both ventricles, and finally, d) the mechanism which keeps papillary muscle fiber loading the same as muscle fiber loading in the cardiac wall.

Transmural course of fiber orientation

The interplay between torsional deformation of the left ventricle and the transmural course of fiber orientation in the wall is a major determinant of the transmural distribution of fiber shortening during the ejection phase. Consider a segment of the wall of the left ventricle in the end-diastolic state (Fig. 5A), and the apical direction oriented to the bottom. In the sub-epicardial layers the fibers are directed obliquely from the upper left to the lower right, in the mid layers approximately circumferentially, and in the subendocardial layers obliquely from the upper right to the lower left.[17] In the case of pure contraction of the ventricle without torsion, the inner circumference shortens considerably more than the outer circumference (Fig. 5B), and as a consequence, the subendocardial muscle fibers shorten much more than the subepicardial ones. However, as indicated in Fig. 5C, in the case of pure torsion without change in cavity volume, subepicardial fibers shorten at the cost of lengthening of the subendocardial fibers, while the length of the fibers in the middle layers remains nearly the same. Precise cancelling of the effects of torsion and shortening on the transmural gradient of muscle fiber shortening occurs only at a specific ratio of shortening to torsion (Fig 5D), in combination with a specific transmural distribution of fiber orientation. For this reason the ratio of shortening to torsion in a left ventricle is practically fixed.

As mentioned above, left ventricular pressure is generated by circumferential stress in the wall. This pressure tends to force the apex from the left ventricle away from the basis which is prevented by axial stresses in the wall. Thus the equilibrium of axial forces in the wall of the left ventricle turns out to be an equilibrium between axial and circumferential stress components in this wall. The resultant fixed ratio of axial stress to circumferential stress puts a restriction on the distribution of fiber orientation in the wall. Obviously, the direction of the fibers can be neither only circumferential nor only from base to apex. A second restraint to the transmural course of fiber orientation is put by the equilibrium of torques in the wall. As a result of this, shear stresses caused by the right handed helical fiber pathways in the subendocardial layers must be compensated by stresses associated with left-handed helical pathways in the subepicardial layers. On the basis of both restraints, and the fact that fiber shortening is the same everywhere in the wall, the transmural course of fiber orientation is calculated. In Fig. 6 the bold solid

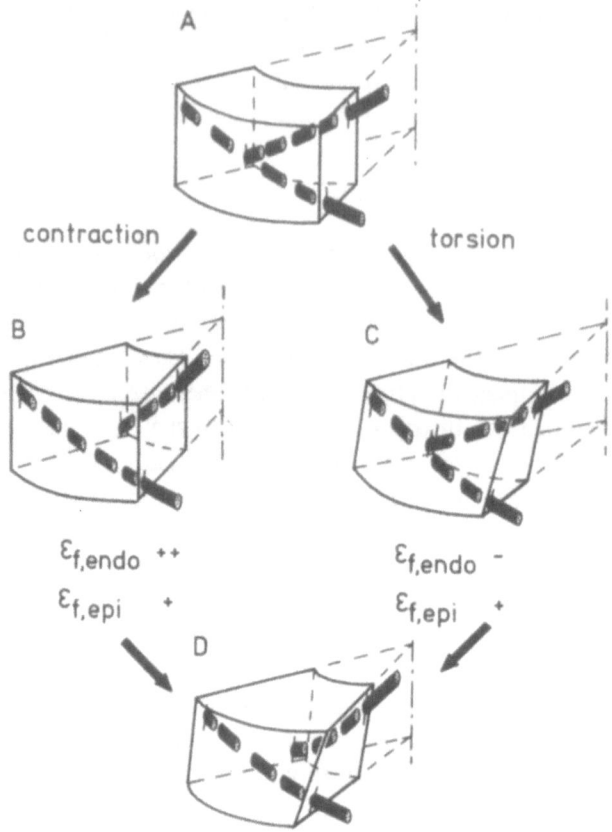

Fig. 5. The effect of torsion and circumferential shortening on the transmural distribution of fiber shortening. Starting from a reference situation (a) a segment of the left ventricular wall might purely shorten circumferentially (b) or purely twist (c). A precise cancelling of transmural differences of fiber shortening in the wall is obtained by weighted combination of both modes of deformation (d). $E_{f,endo}$ and $E_{f,epi}$ denote subendocardial and subepicardial fiber shortening, respectively.

lines represent the fiber angle as a function of the distance from the endocardium at an amount of fiber shortening (20%) required for that particular heart beat on the basis that the total amount of stroke work produced by the muscle is equal to hemodynamic stroke work. The two curves satisfy the restriction of 20% fiber shortening. However, the equilibrium of torques requires positive and negative fiber angles, which leads to the use of the upper curve. In order to keep the axial stress component sufficiently high and close to the epicardium a jump from one characteristic to the other is made. The accuracy by which the fiber angle is determined, is indicated by the shaded area denoting the region where fiber shortening is in between 18% and 22% shortening. Thus it can be seen that close to the

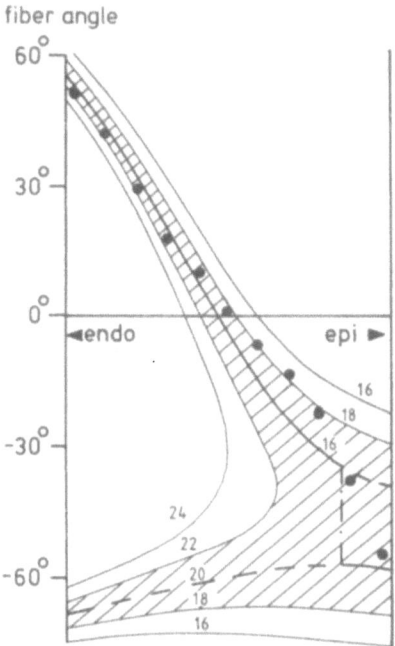

Fig. 6. Angle between muscle fiber direction and equator as a function of depth in the wall. The bold, solid line represents the calculated curve with 20% fiber shortening. In the shaded area fiber shortening ranges from 18% to 22%. Thus in the subepicardial layers, the fiber angle is less critical than in the subendocardial layers. The dots represent experimental data by Streeter et al.[25]

epicardium fiber orientation is not critical. The dots represent the data found in experiments on canine hearts by Streeter et al.[23] and fit quite accurately in the shaded area.

Relation of left ventricular pressure and volume to fiber stress and sarcomere length

Because muscle fiber load is the same everywhere, a search for a direct and simple relationship between hemodynamic quantities like pressures and flows and quantities related to muscular mechanics like stress and sarcomere length is made. In the model, empirically the following relation between sarcomere length (L_s) and left ventricular cavity volume (V_{lv}) was found to hold for a wide range of preload (end)dystolic volume), afterload (end-diastolic aortic pressure) and contractility levels:

$$L_s = L_{so} \cdot (1 + 3 \cdot V_{lv}/V_w)^{1/3} \tag{1}$$

where L_{so} = extrapolated sarcomere length at zero cavity volume and

V_w = left ventricular wall volume. Using the property that hemodynamic pumping energy equals the energy generated by cardiac muscle tissue in the wall, the following relation between cavity pressure (P_{lv}) and muscle fiber stress (S_f) can be derived[12] from Eq (1):

$$S_f = P_{lv} \cdot (1 + 3V_{lv}/V_w) \tag{2}$$

Eq (1) and (2) represent a simple set of equations, describing the relationship between left ventricular volume and pressure, muscle fiber stress and sarcomere length. Unlike in other, previously described relation between cavity pressure and wall stress,[9,24] in our relations, no parameters describing the shape of the left ventricle are found in these equations. In an attempt to find out, whether Eq (1) and (2) apply to other geometries than the cylinder, a more general equation was derived between left ventricular pressure increment (d P_{lv}) and wall volume increment (d V_{wi}), being valid for a cylindrical as well as a spherical shell (cf. Appendix):

$$d\,P_{lv} = (S_f/3V) \cdot d\,V_{wi} \tag{3}$$

where V represents the volume enclosed by the shell. Integration of Eq 3 over the wall, taking V being equal to the sum of cavity volume and enclosed wall volume, finally results in

$$P_{lv} = (S_f/3)\,\ln(1 + V_w/V_{lv}) \tag{4}$$

Fig. 7 shows a variant of Eq (4), expressing the ratio of fiber stress to left ventricular volume as a function of the ratio of left ventricular volume as a function of the ratio of left ventricular cavity volume to wall volume. This equation is different from Eq 2, but as can be seen from Fig. 7 the difference between both curves is only in the order of 7% in the normal range of left ventricular volumes (0.3 V_{lv}/V_w 0.6). Application of the transformation procedure, used to obtain Eq (2) from Eq (1), in a backward fashion to Eq (4) reveals for the relation between sarcomere length and left ventricular volume

$$L_s/L_{So} = [(1 + x)^{1 + x}/x^x]^{1/3} \tag{5}$$

with $x = V_{lv}/V_w$. As shown in Fig. 8 this more complicated, but this more exact equation differs only slightly from the simpler Eq (1). Thus it is found that the relation between left ventricular pressure, volume, fiber stress, and sarcomere length is the same for a sphere and a cylinder. The most exact description is made by Eq (4) and (5), but for simplicity Eq (1) and (2) may be used as a good approximation.

In Fig. 9 stress–sarcomere length loops are shown, which correspond to the pressure-volume loops shown in Fig 4. Qualitatively, these curves are not much different from such loops obtained by other formulas for wall stress,

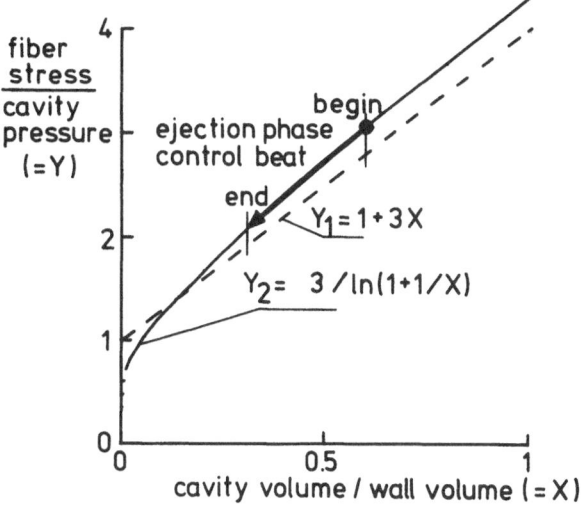

Fig. 7. Muscle fiber stress, normalized to left ventricular pressure, is plotted as a function of left ventricular cavity volume, as normalized to wall volume. The solid line represents the more exact relation, and the broken line a reasonably accurate, but simpler description.

but quantitatively there is a difference. Our equation reveals muscle fiber stresses approximately 1.5 to 2.0 times higher than with conventional equations.[9,24] In a regular cardiac beat, during mid-ejection the ratio of left ventricular cavity volume to wall volume is in the order of 0.4. Using Eq (2), at a peak left ventricular pressure of 16 kPa ($\sim$ = 120 mmHg), muscle fiber stress is calculated to be 35 kPas (= 3.5 gr mm^{-2}). The latter value is close

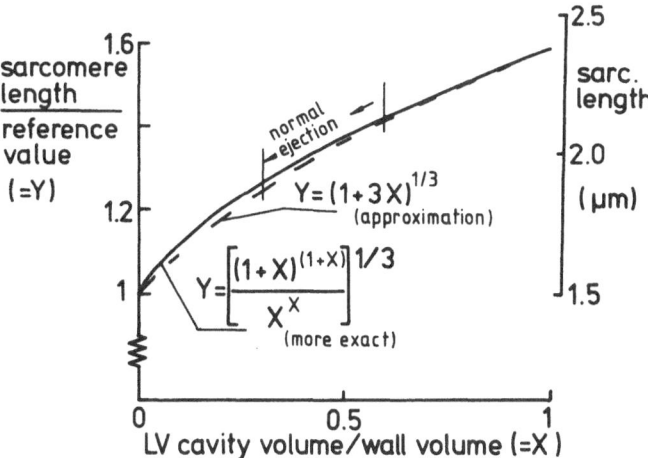

Fig. 8. Sarcomere length, as normalized to extrapolated sarcomere length at zero cavity volume, plotted as a function of normalized cavity volume. The difference between the simple relation (broken line) and the exact, but more complex relation (solid line) is marginal.

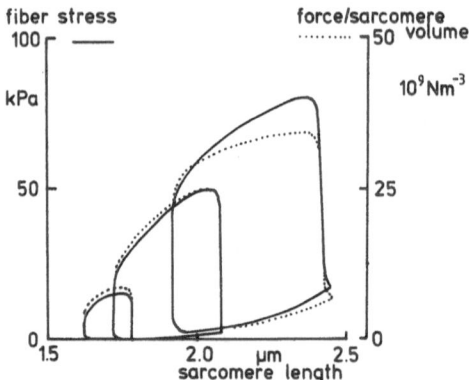

Fig. 9. Muscle fiber stress–sarcomere length loops (solid lines), as associated with the pressure–volume loops in Fig. 4. The dotted lines represent the relation between muscle fiber force, as normalized to sarcomere volume, and sarcomere length.

to the isotonic stress load, used in *in vitro* experiments on isolated cardiac muscle generating mechanical work optimally. During isovolumic contraction of the left ventricle, induced by aortic occlusion, cavity pressure may rise to 35 kPa (= 262 mmHg). Assuming, the ratio of cavity volume to wall volume in such a non-ejecting beat equals 0.55, muscle fiber stress is calculated to be approximately 93 kPa (= 9.3 gr mm^{-2}). The latter value is also close to the values of muscle stress obtained during isometric contraction. Application of Eq (4) to the intact left ventricle results in values for muscle fiber stress, which are in close agreement with the findings obtained in experiments performed on isolated cardiac muscle.

Fig. 9 also shows muscle fiber force as normalized to sarcomere volume (= fiber stress/sarcomere length) as a function of sarcomere length. The advantage of using this quantity is that it forms a pair with sarcomere length the mutual product of which is energy per unit of tissue volume. So the areas of the dotted loops in Fig. 9 represent stroke energy per unit of tissue volume. These loops may be compared with $P_{lv} - V_{lv}$ loops of the left ventricle. Moreover, in isolated muscle preparations, muscle volume is constant during contraction, so the force measured is proportional to normalized fiber force, without the need of a correction due to thickening of the muscle during contraction. Calculation of fiber stress needs such a correction.

The ratio of right to left ventricular weight

Using our hypothesis on homogeneity of muscle fiber stress and shortening, generated mechanical power is proportional to the weight of the muscle involved. Observing the cross-section of the heart (Fig. 10), the left ventricle

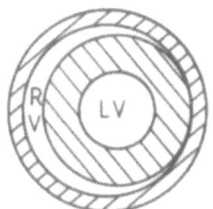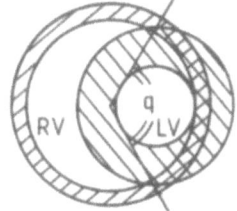

Fig. 10. Schematic representation of the short-axis cross-section of the heart. The heart is conceived to be an inner wall, enclosed by an outer wall (left panel). Shifting of the inner cavity to the left side of the heart (right panel) results in a reasonably realistic representation. LV–left ventricle, RV–right ventricle, q = sector angle of the outer wall located with in the left ventricular wall.

is thick-walled and circular. The right ventricular cavity is segment-like with a much thinner wall. The left panel of Fig 10 shows how this structure can be interpreted. The left ventricular cavity is enclosed by an inner wall. This system, together with the right ventricular wall, is enclosed by the outer wall. During systole the inner wall ejects one stroke volume (V_{stroke}), and the outer wall the sum of the stroke volumes of both left and right ventricle. On average, both stroke volumes are the same, so outer wall stroke volume is twice as much as inner wall stroke volume. Furthermore, systolic left ventricular pressure is approximately 4 times as high as right ventricular pressure. Thus the ratio of outer wall stroke work (E_{outer}) to inner wall stroke work (E_{inner}) is approximately:

$$E_{outer}/E_{inner} = 2P_{lv} \cdot V_{stroke}/(P_{lv} - P_{rv}) \cdot V_{stroke} = 0.67$$

The right panel of Fig. 10 shows a more realistic shape of the cross)section. The free wall of the right ventricle is indicated to be a fraction of the outer wall, depending on the opening angle (q) between the junctions of left and right ventricular free wall. Based on three experimental measurements on two-dimensional echocardiographic images, this angle was approximately 120°. The mass of part of the outer wall spanning the angle (q) is added to the left ventricular wall. Thus, the ratio of mass of the right ventricular free wall (M_{rvfw}) to that of the left ventricle with septum ($M_{lv + sept}$) is calculated to be:

$$M_{rvfw}/M_{lv + sept} = 0.67(1-120°/360°)/1 + 0.67 \cdot 120°/36° = 0.36$$

As shown in Fig. 11, in experiments performed on 12 canine hearts this ratio was found to be 0.35 ± 0.03 (mean ± sd), which is close to the calculated value. Furthermore, the standard deviation of this ratio is quite small, suggesting the presence of some mechanism keeping this ratio within a small range. As pointed out above, keeping fiber stress constant everywhere could be such a mechanism.

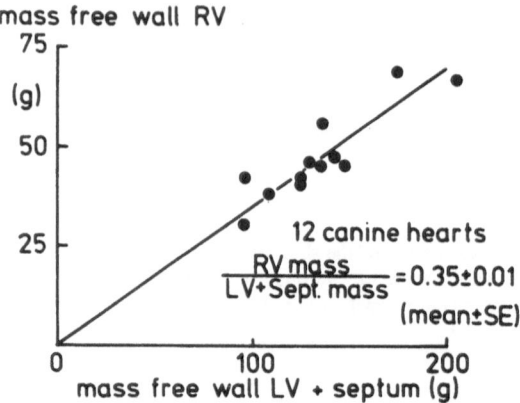

Fig. 11. Experimental data obtained from 12 canine hearts. Mass of the free wall of the right ventricle is plotted as a function of the added mass of the free wall of the left ventricle and septum. The experimentally found value for the slope is close to the theoretical estimate (0.36).

The mitral valve – papillary muscle system

The anatomy of the mitral valve is an important determinant of the mechanical loading of this valve and the papillary muscles. The mitral valve orifice (Fig. 1) is surrounded by an annular ring, bordering the contracting basal region of the anterolateral left ventricular free wall for one half, and a passive fibrous basal sheet which covers the top of the left ventricular cavity for the other half. The leaflets of the valve hinge to the annular ring. The tips of the leaflets are attached to the chordae tendineae, which in turn are connected to the papillary muscle. Thus the force to be born by the papillary muscles is a result of tension in the mitral valve leaflets.

During systole, left ventricular pressure increases resulting in an increase of papillary muscle force. If the geometry of the mitral valve would not change during the ejection phase, papillary muscle force would be proportional to left ventricular pressure. As a result, at the end of the ejection phase papillary muscle stress would not have dropped sufficiently to follow fiber stress in the other parts of the cardiac muscle (Fig. 2). However, mitral valve geometry varies as a result of the decrease of base to apex distance and left ventricular inner radius, during the ejection phase. The radii of curvature of the mitral valve leaflets decrease, causing a decrease in leaflet stress according to Laplace's law. The change in mitral geometry appears to be tuned in such a way that the decrease of papillary muscle stress matches the decrease of muscle fiber stress in the other structures of the left ventricle quite precisely (Fig. 2). The latter model finding agrees with experimental findings reported by Salisbury et al.[25] They measured chordae tendineae force during the cardiac cycle, and found a large decrease of this force during the ejection phase, while left ventricular pressures changed only moderately.

Conclusion

When postulating muscle fiber stress to be the same everywhere in the heart, a mathematical representation of the mechanics of the left ventricle can be found, which satisfies the related hypothesis. Furthermore, reasonable agreement between mathematical predictions and experimental findings is found with respect to: 1) the amount of torsion and circumferential shortening of the left ventricle, as well as the ratio between these quantities, 2) the transmural course of muscle fiber orientation in the wall of the left ventricle, 3) the quantitative values of muscle fiber stress in the heart, as compared to experimental findings on isolated cardiac muscle, 4) the ratio of weight between left and right ventricular wall, and 5) the time course of papillary muscle force, being related to the geometry of the base – mitral valve – chordae tendineae – papillary muscle system.

Appendix

Relation between fiber stress and pressure in a thin-walled cavity

Consider a thin-walled body. Along orthogonal coordinates x and y, for the normal stress components S_{xx} and S_{yy} s a result of a fiber stress S_f in the wall it holds

$$S_{xx} = S_f \cos^2 p; \; S_{yy} = S_f \sin^2 p \tag{A1}$$

where p is the angle between the fiber direction and the X-coordinate. So, for the sum of these components it holds:

$$S_{xx} + S_{yy} = S_f \tag{A2}$$

In a cylinder with radius r, wall thickness h, length l and internal pressure P, for the circumferential and axial wall stress components it holds, respectively:

$$S_{cc} = P \cdot r/h; \; S_{zz} = P \cdot r/2h \tag{A3}$$

and for a sphere it holds:

$$S_{cc} = S_{zz} = P \cdot r/2h \tag{A4}$$

For the ratio of cavity volume to wall volume of the cylinder and the sphere it holds, respectively:

$$V_c/V_{wc} = r/2h; \quad V_c/V_{ws} = r/3h \tag{A5}$$

Combination of Eq (A2), (A3) and (A5) for the cylinder, and Eq (A2), (A4) and (A5) for the sphere both result in the same general equation

$$P/S_f = V_c/3V_w \tag{A6}$$

which is equivalent to Eq (3).

References

1. Janz RF and Grimm AF (1972). Finite element model for the mechanical behavior of the left ventricle. Circ Res 30: 224–252.
2. Pao YC, Robb RA and Ritman EL (1976). Plain-strain finite-element analysis of reconstructed diastolic left ventricular cross-section. Ann Biomed Eng 4: 232–249.
3. Yettram AL, Vinson CA and Gibson DG (1983). Effect of myocardial fiber architecture on the behavior of the human left ventricle in diastole. J Biomed Eng 5: 321–328.
4. Feith TS (1979). Diastolic pressure–volume relations and distribution of pressure and fiber extension across the wall of a model left ventricle. Biophys J 28: 143–166.
5. Meier GD, Ziskin MC and Bove AA (1982). Helical fibers in myocardium. Am J Physiol 243: H1–H12.
6. Streeter DD, Spotnitz HM, Patel DP, Ross J and Sonnenblick EH (1969). Fiber orientation in the canine left ventricle during diastole and systole. Circ Res 24: 339–347.
7. Back L (1977). Left ventricular wall and fluid dynamics of cardiac contraction. Mathemat Biosc 36: 257–297.
8. Beyar R and Sideman S (1984). Model for left ventricular contraction combining the force length velocity relationship with the time varying elastance theory. Biophys J 45: 1167–1177.
9. Mirsky I (1969). Left ventricular stresses in the intact human heart. Biophys J 9: 189–208.
10. Weber KT, Janicki SJ and Heffner LL (1976). Left ventricular force–length relation of isovolumic and ejecting contraction. Am J Physiol 231: 337–343.
11. Arts T, Veentra PC and Reneman RS (1979). A model of the mechanics of the left ventricle. Ann Biomed Eng 7: 299–318.
12. Arts T, Veentra PC and Reneman RS (1982). Epicardial deformation and left ventricular wall mechanics during ejection in the dog. Am J Physiol 243: H379–H390.
13. Chadwick RS (1982). Mechanics of the left ventricle. Biophys J 39: 212–220.
14. Bache RJ, McHale PA and Greenfield JC (1977). Transmural myocardial perfusion during restricted coronary inflow in the awake dog. Am J Physiol 232: H645–H651.
15. Prinzen FW (1982). Gradients in myocardial bloodflow, metabolism and mechanics across the ischemic left ventricular wall. Thesis, University of Limburg, Maastricht, The Netherlands.
16. Bache RJ and Schwartz JS (1983). Myocardial bloodflow during exercise after gradual coronary occlusion in the dog. Am J Physiol 245: H131–H138.
17. Guasp FT (1973). The cardiac muscle. Ed. Torroba, Madric Spain.
18. Westerhof N, Elzinga G and Van den Bosch GC (1973). Influence of central and peripheral changes on the hydraulic input impedance of the systemic arterial tree. Med Biol Eng 11: 710–722.
19. Nolan SP (1976). The normal mitral valve: patterns of instantaneous mitral valve flow and the atrial contribution to ventricular filling. In: The mitral valve, D. Kalmanson (ed.), Publ Sci Group Inc, Massachusetts, pp 137–143.
20. Yellin EL, Peskin C, Koeningsberg M, Matsumoto M, Laniado S, McQueen D, Shore D and Frater RWM (1981). Mechanisms of mitral valve motion during diastole.

21. Suga H, Hisano R, Goto Y, Yamada O and Igarashi Y (1981). Effect of positive inotropic agents on the relation between oxygen consumption and systolic pressure volume area in canine left ventricle. Circ Res 53: 306–318.
22. Arts T, Veentra PC and Reneman RS (1979). A model of the mechanics of the left ventricle. Ann Biomed Eng 7: 299–318.
23. Streeter DD, Vaisjnav RN, Patel DJ, Spotnitz HM, Ross J and Sonnenblick EH (1970). Stress distribution in the canine left ventricle during diastole and systole. Biophys J 10: 345–363.
24. McHale PA and Greenfield JC (1973). Evaluation of several geometric models for estimation of left ventricular circumferential wall stress. Circ Res 33: 303–312.
25. Salisbury PF, Cross CE and Rieben PA (1963). Chordae tendineae tension. Am J Physiol 205: 385–392.

9. Cardiac Pump Function and Ventricular Dimensions

G. ELZINGA, G.J. VAN DER HORN & N. WESTERHOF

Laboratorium voor Fysiologie, Vrije Universiteit, Amsterdam, The Netherlands

Abstract

The size of the heart depends on the size of the animal because ventricular dimensions are related to the pressure and flow the ventricle has to generate. This principle holds true also within a given animal. Geometry and size of the heart change with a long term increase in pressure (concentric hypertrophy) and a dimensional change is also seen with a systematic increase in cardiac output (eccentric hypertrophy).

Experimental evidence suggests that the circulation is controlled to keep the ventricle at optimum power output. In this chapter it is argued that this circulatory control principle may be related to the occurrence of different types of dimensional change, such as concentric and eccentric hypertrophy.

Introduction

It is well known that the size of the heart bears a close relationship to the size of the animal. It is often said that the cause for this relationship is to be found in the absolute differences in cardiac output between species, which, in turn, reflects the dependency of the total amount of energy used on animal size. Also, within the same species ventricular dimensions appear to depend on the average level of energy turnover. When, for instance, metabolic activity increases as occurs in athletes performing duration exercise, heart size increases.

The metabolic requirements of the body, and thus cardiac output, is not the sole determinant of ventricular dimensions. For instance changes in circulatory control leading to high blood pressure also lead to changes in ventricular geometry. The dimensional changes which occur in such a situation differ from those seen with an increase in cardiac output. In the latter case the ventricular lumen increases in size and a moderate wall thickening

H.E.D.J. ter Keurs and M.I.M. Noble (eds), Starling's Law of the Heart Revisited. ISBN 978-94-010-7084-3
© 1988, Kluwer Academic Publishers, Dordrecht

occurs: eccentric hypertrophy. In the former case no enlargement of the ventricular lumen takes place but wall thickness increases markedly: concentric hypertrophy.

Thus changes in circulatory demand leading to hypertrophy go together with functional changes of the ventricular pump. In the present chapter we discuss some principles which may be involved in the pump function changes, occurring with different types of hypertrophy. The ideas developed here may be relevant in particular in the case of "physiological" hypertrophy.[1]

Matching

It has been suggested that hypertrophy is due to an increase in workload on the heart. Such statements are more often than not made in the belief that an increase in workload necessarily implies an increase in cardiac energy turnover. However, this need not be the case and it is necessary for the present discussion to be clear about the precise relation between ventricular pump function, work output, and energy turnover. Figure 1 shows these relationships for the left ventricle of a cat.[2] In the top panel the pump function graph is shown, i.e. the inverse relationship between ventricular output and mean pressure obtained by changes in the arterial load at a given end-diastolic volume, heart rate and inotropic state. The mean external power delivered by the ventricle is obtained by integrating the instantaneous product of pressure and flow and varies along the pump function graph in a parabola-like manner (middle panel). Oxygen consumption (which is, for the aerobic conditions under which these data were obtained, directly proportional to total energy turnover (bottom panel)), is the highest for the highest pressure, and thus the lowest output. From the shape of the curves in the two lower panels it can already be concluded that the relationship between power production and energy turnover is complex. An increase in work output of the ventricle does not therefore always imply an increase in the energy turnover and the two certainly do not change in proportion.

When ventricular pump function changes, as is the case with changes in end-diastolic volume, inotropic state, heart rate and ventricular dimensions, the situation becomes more complex and the relative directions of changes in power output and energy turnover are difficult to predict without more specific information. Knowledge about the "working point", i.e. the pressure and flow value generated by the ventricle at the prevailing arterial load on the graphs shown in Figure 1 is therefore required.

In 1964, Wilcken et al.[3] found in intact conscious resting dogs that the left ventricle to operated at peak power output. Their results, shown in Fig. 2, form a limited portion of the curve shown in Fig. 1b for isolated cat hearts.

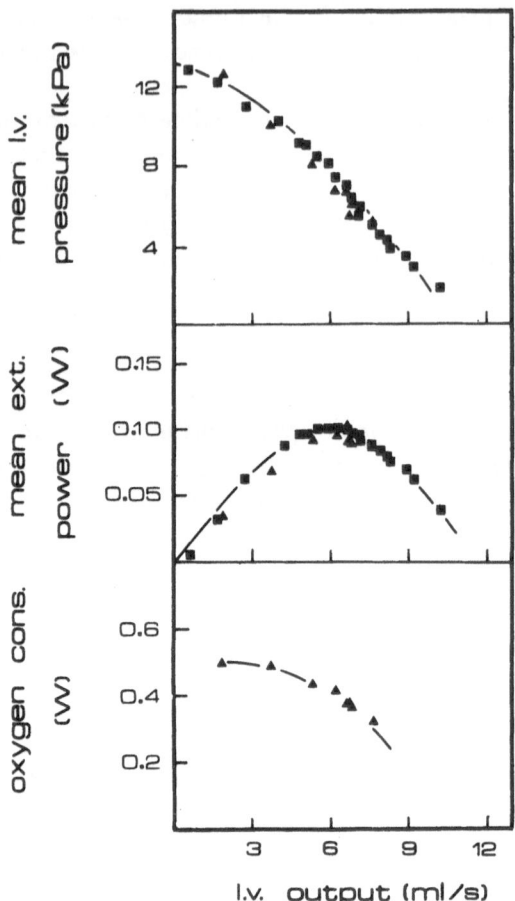

Fig. 1. Mean left ventricular pressure (top panel), mean external power (middle panel) and oxygen consumption (bottom panel) plotted as a function of left ventricular output. The data were obtained from an isolated ejecting cat heart preparation through variations of the arterial load while end-diastolic volume, heart rate and inotropic state were constant.[2]

They concluded that the working point of the in situ left ventricle of the dog was at the point of optimum external power.

This observation led to the idea that the circulation is controlled as to maintain external power transfer from ventricle to arterial system; this condition is known in electrical circuits as impedance matching.[4] Although the situation in the circulation is not the same as that in simple electrical analogs, (and therefore serious questions about the validity of the matching concept for the relation between ventricle and arterial system require an answer), work matching is regularly used to indicate the general notion that the hemodynamic properties of ventricle and arterial system are related to one another.

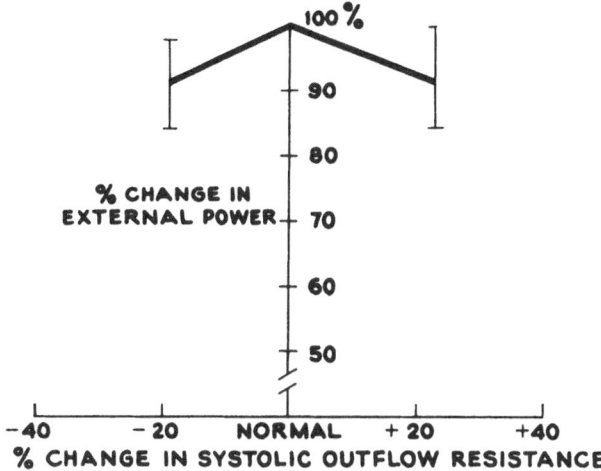

Fig. 2. In the conscious resting dog sudden alterations in arterial load revealed that external power decreased with an increase as well as with a decrease of the load. Note that now a measure of resistance instead of output is plotted on the abscissa (data from Wilcken et al.[3]).

The idea that the hemodynamic properties of the heart and the arterial system are adapted to each other is not new. In 1935 Broemser[5] claimed already that the duration of the cardiac systole and the properties of the arterial system were designed to optimize stroke volume. Later O'Rourke[6] and also Milnor[7] postulated that the minimum found by some investigators in the arterial input impedance provided an opportunity for the heart to pump at a frequency which would result in minimal (oscillatory) energy loss. However, the use of work matching to indicate the relationship between heart rate and arterial load addresses a different aspect of circulatory control. In this chapter we will not deal with that, but discuss only some possible consequences of the apparent property of the circulatory control systems to keep the ventricular pump at optimum power output. Before doing that we will first present experimental evidence illustrating the occurrence of that property.

Experimental evidence

The findings of Wilcken et al.[3] that in the resting conscious dog the left ventricle operates at peak power output made further investigation necessary to obtain sufficient experimental support support for the idea that the occurrence of this specific position of the ventricle on the power output graph (Fig. 1, middle panel) is the result of an integrated circulatory control mechanism. In particular, experiments were required to test aspects of the concept of a feedback system that keeps the heart at optimum power output; this raises questions about the likelihood of power receptors and about the complexity of the information required in such a system to function properly.

Making use of isolated cat right ventricles Piene and Sund[8,9] found that maximum external power was generated for flows and pressures in the "normal" or "physiological" range. Similar results were obtained by Suna-gawa et al.[10,11] for isolated canine left ventricles. Elzinga et al.[2,12] showed that this held true as well for the isolated cat left ventricle. They also demon-strated that the optimum power output of left and right ventricle, which differed in magnitude by a factor 5, were found at approximately the same cardiac output.

The position of the ventricle on the pump function graph (Fig. 1, top panel) and therefore on the power output graph depends on the properties of the heart and the properties of the arterial system. This implies that in vivo control systems of both these parts of the circulation must be involved if the finding of Wilcken et al.[3] (see above) is interpreted as evidence for the existence of a feedback system controlling the circulation. Experimental support obtained from isolated preparations can therefore provide no more than indirect evidence in support of that concept.

To obtain more direct evidence for the existence of this specific property of the circulatory control systems, in vivo experiments have been done. In open thorax cats under anaesthesia the finding of Wilcken et al.[3] was confirmed by van der Horn et al.[13] These investigators also attempted, in the same preparation, to change the experimental conditions such that the ventricle would no longer operate at optimum work output. Moderate changes in he level of anaesthesia, heart rate and circulatory filling caused changes in ventricular pump function but the ventricle remained at the (also altered) optimum power output.[13] Only with noradrenaline infusions was the working point of the ventricle no longer maintained at the optimum power output.[14] Myhre and Piene[15] studied open thorax dogs under anaesthesia and found under control conditions that again the ventricle operated at optimum power output. Injection of large microspheres to occlude coronary vessels and cause deterioration of cardiac function drove the ventricle away from this position.

Apart from Wilcken et al.[3] no complete experiments have been reported on conscious animals, although Kuwait de Jonge[16] provided indirect evidence that in the running dog the working point is no longer maintained at optimum power output, as was found at rest by Wilcken et al.[3]

Therefore from the experimental evidence available no definite conclusions can be drawn but the findings so far may be interpreted to suggest that an integrated circulatory control mechanism exists which keeps (within hemody-namic limits) the left ventricle at optimum power output. With severe changes in the hemodynamic conditions the optimum power output is no longer maintained and a "mismatch" occurs between ventricle and arterial system. Taking this notion, which is not yet sufficiently supported, as a working hypothesis we will now discuss the pump function changes required to restore a situation of "mismatch" resulting from a pressure and volume overload into a "matched" situation.

Postulate

Before discussing the pump function changes which may be expected from cardiac adaptation following a mismatch due to pressure and volume over-load, it is helpful to look once more at the pump function graph (Fig. 1, top panel). The pressure used in this relationship is the mean pressure in the left ventricle. Since the myocardial cells form the basic elements building the cardiac pump, left ventricular pressure bears an instantaneous and direct relationship to the forces produced by the myocardial fibers.

When we look at the other side of the aortic valve, it is well known that the ratio of mean (aortic) pressure (minus venous pressure) and flow represents the peripheral resistance. It has been shown by van der Horn et al.,[13] that a proportionality exists between mean aortic pressure and mean ventricular pressure. On the basis of this finding the pump function graph and peripheral resistance can be equally well expressed in terms of mean aortic or mean ventricular pressure if the proportionality constant is known. This knowledge is very convenient because it allows plotting of the pump function graph and the peripheral resistance in the same diagram (Fig. 3).

If we now turn to the question, "In what way can the ventricle adapt to an increase in arterial blood pressure (hypertension) to turn the "mismatch" resulting initially from that hemodynamic change into a "matched" situation"?, we can make use of the schematic diagram shown in Fig. 4. It is known that with hypertension cardiac output remains normal. In the pressure flow diagram the working point of the left ventricle therefore moves upwards with an increase in peripheral resistance. The change in slope of the line through the origin and the working point corresponds to the increase in peripheral resistance. Since pressure increases and flow remains the same the new working point cannot be located on the initial pump function graph. The new pump function graph, which fulfills the requirement for the ventricle to remain at peak power output, has the same intercept on the abscissa but a much higher intercept on the ordinate.

An attempt is made in Fig. 5 to predict what would happen to cardiac pump function in the case of volume overload, if circulatory control tries to maintain the ventricle at optimum power output. With volume overload cardiac output is increased but mean blood pressure remains about the same.

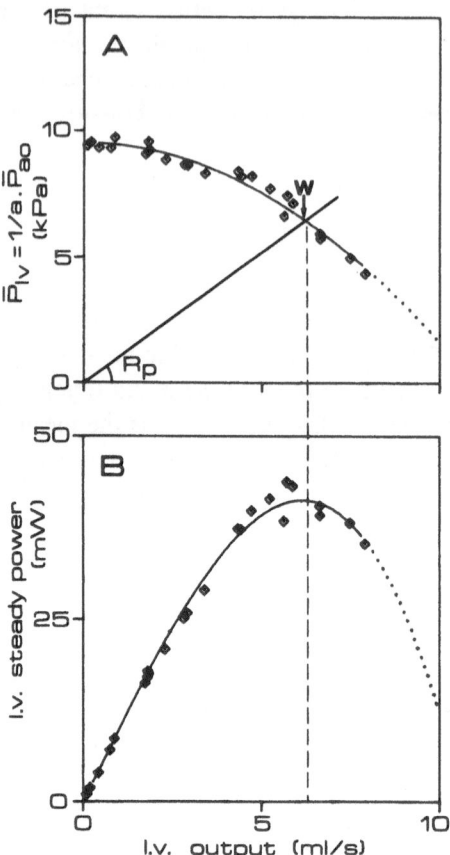

Fig. 3. Because a proportional relationship was found between mean aortic and mean left ventricular pressure, the slope of the line drawn through the origin and the working point is proportional to the peripheral resistance (Rp). In the example given here the working point is found at the same output as the point of optimum power output. The results were obtained in an open thorax cat.[13]

Therefore the working point moves to the right (Fig. 5). This cannot happen without a change in pump function because then pressure has to decline with an increase in output. There are, in principle, an infinite number of positions this graph can have in order to incorporate the new working point. However, there is only a single pump function graph which would do so and bring at the same time the working point back to the optimum of the new power output graph. That pump function graph would have the same intercept on the ordinate while the intercept on the abscissa would be much higher.

When we now look at the changes in ventricular dimensions which occur with pressure and volume overload (Fig. 6) we see that concentric hypertrophy is characterized by a selective thickening of the ventricular wall. This development increases the pressure generating capacity, but as the ventricular

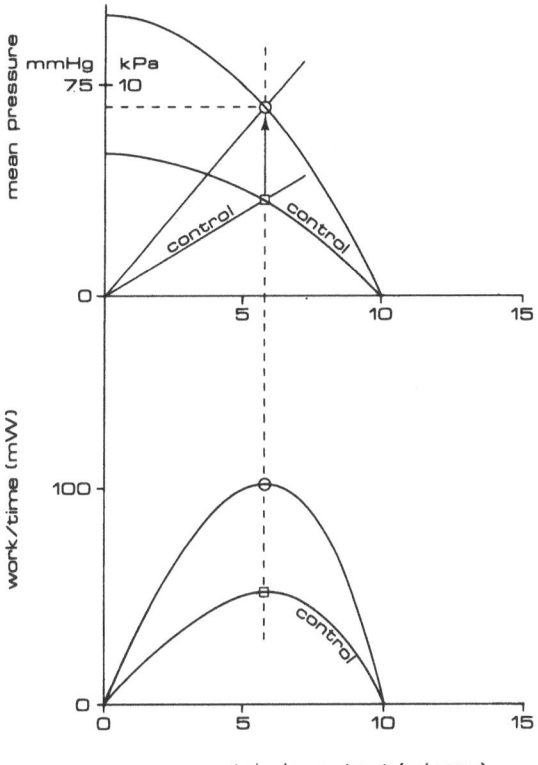

Fig. 4. When at a given ventricular output, arterial pressure increases systematically, (i.e. an increase in peripheral resistance), hypertrophy occurs and causes a change in ventricular pump function. The new cardiac pump function curve rotates around the intercept on the abscissa when the working point remains at optimum power output.

lumen does not change the maximum output at a given heart rate remains the same. This type of change corresponds to the change of ventricular pump function required to bring the workpoint back to the position of optimum power output (Fig. 4).

Eccentric hypertrophy resulting from a volume overload (Fig. 6) is characterized by an increase in size of the lumen. Wall thickness increases to some extent. This dimensional change would occur if the heart had to acquire a pump function graph, as described above, with an increased value for the intercept on the flow axis and the same mean isometric pressure. The increase in wall thickness in the case of eccentric hypertrophy would not lead to an increased capacity to generate pressure, but is necessary to compensate for the increase in lumen radius (wall thickness over radius about the same as for normal hearts).

Apart from these two types of hypertrophy resulting from clearly defined hemodynamic changes, a third type is often encountered for which the cause

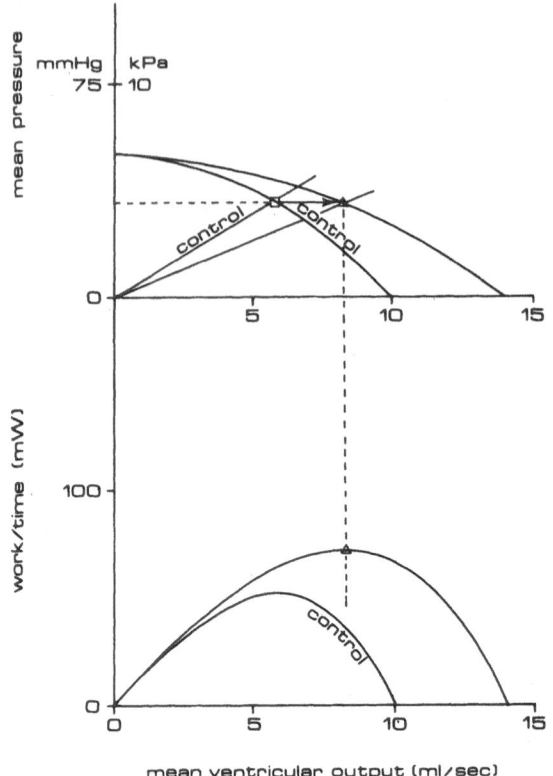

Fig. 5. When at a given arterial pressure, systemic increase in output occurs, (i.e. a decrease in peripheral resistance), hypertrophy results and ventricular pump function changes. The new pump function graph rotates around the intercept on the ordinate when the working point remains at optimum power output.

is much less clear: idiopathic hypertrophy. Although difficult, it is not impossible to bring the occurrence of this type of hypertrophy in agreement with the postulate, that we deal here with an integrated control mechanism designed to keep the ventricle at the peak of the power output curve. Disturbances in the feedback loopsettings could in principle lead to hypertrophy without prior changes in pressure or output.

So far no experiments have been done to falsify the hypothesis that the integrated circulatory control system is designed to keep the ventricle at peak power output and that this mechanism determines the occurrence of the different types of hypertrophy described in the literature. However, there is one small piece of experimental evidence which is worthwhile mentioning:

Before birth, the shape and function of the right ventricle differ from that after birth. Although we have no information regarding the working point of the right ventricle on the power output graph before and directly after birth,

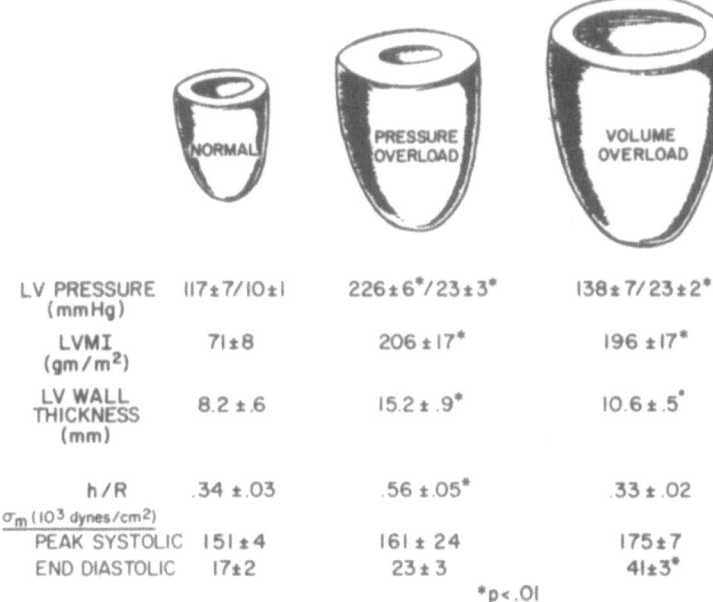

	NORMAL	PRESSURE OVERLOAD	VOLUME OVERLOAD
LV PRESSURE (mmHg)	117±7/10±1	226±6*/23±3*	138±7/23±2*
LVMI (gm/m²)	71±8	206±17*	196±17*
LV WALL THICKNESS (mm)	8.2±.6	15.2±.9*	10.6±.5*
h/R	.34±.03	.56±.05*	.33±.02
σ_m (10³ dynes/cm²) PEAK SYSTOLIC	151±4	161±24	175±7
END DIASTOLIC	17±2	23±3	41±3*

*p<.01

Fig. 6. Left ventricular (LV) pressure, left ventricular mass index (LVMI), wall thickness, ratio of wall thickness to radius (h/R) at end diastole, and meridional left ventricular wall stress (m) in patients with normal hearts compared to those with chronic left ventricular pressure overload or volume overload. Only patients with chronic left ventricular pressure or volume overload who were well compensated and had no depression of systolic function (LV ejection fraction) were included. From Grossman et al.[17]

we know that the hemodynamic changes lead eventually to the situation that the right and left ventricle are operating at optimum work output at the same flow.[2,12] This can be regarded as indirect evidence in support of the hypothesis put forward.

References

1. Bishop SP (1983). Ultrastructure of the myocardium in physiologic and pathologic hypertrophy in experimental animals. In: Perspectives in Cardiovascular Research, Vol. 7, Myocardial Hypertrophy and Failure, NR Alpert (ed.), Raven Press, New York, p. 127–147.
2. Elzinga G and Westerhof N (1980a). Pump function of the feline left heart: changes with heart rate and its bearing to the energy balance. Cardiovasc Res 14: 81–92.
3. Wilcken DEL, Charlier AA, Hoffman JIE and Guz A (1964). Effects of alterations in aortic impedence on the performance of the ventricles. Circ Res 14: 283–293.
4. Van Valkenburg ME (1964). Network analysis. Prentice Hall, Inc., Englewood Cliffs, New Jersey (2nd edition).
5. Broemser Ph (1935). Ueber die optimalen Beziehungen zwischen Herztatigkeit und physikalisaachen Konstanten des Gefasssystems. Z Biol 96: 11–10.
6. O'Rourke MF (1965). Pressure and flow in arteries. MD Thesis, University of Sydney, Australia.

7. Milnor WR (1979). Aortic wavelength as a determinant of the relation between heart rate and body size in mammals. Am J Physiol 237: R3–R6.
8. Piene H and Sund T (1979). Flow and power output of right ventricle facing load with variable input impedence. Am J Physiol 237: H125–H160.
9. Piene H and Sund T (1982). Does pulmonary input impedence constitute the optimum load for the right ventricle Am J Physiol 242: H154–H160.
10. Sunagawa K, Maughan WL and Sagawa K (1983a). Left ventricular interaction with the arterial loading system. Ann Biomed Eng 11: 52.
11. Sunagawa K, Maughan WL, Burkhoff D and Sagawa K (1983b). Left ventricular interaction with arterial load studied in isolated canine ventricle. Am J Physiol 245: H773–H780.
12. Elzinga G, Piene H and De Jong JP (1980b). Left and right ventricular pump function and the consequences of having two pumps in one heart. Circ Res 46: 564–574.
13. Van Den Horn GJ, Westerhof N and Elzinga G (1985). Optimal power generation by the left ventricle: a study in the anesthetized open thorax cat. Circ Res 56: 252–261.
14. Van Den Horn GJ, Westerhof N and Elzinga G (1986). The feline left ventricle does not always operate at optimum power output. Am J Physiol, In Press.
15. Myhre L, Johansen A, Bjornstat J and Piene H (1986). The effect of contractility and preload on matching between the canine left ventricle and afterload. Circ 73: 161–171.
16. Kiewiet De Jonge M (1981). Circulatory effects of myocardial infarction at rest and during exercise. PhD Thesis, Amsterdam.
17. Grossman W, Jones D and McLaurin LP (1975). Wall stress patterns of hypertrophy. J Clin Invest 56: 56–64.

10. The Pressure–Volume Relationship of the Intact Heart

MARK I.M. NOBLE

King Edward VII Hospital, Midhurst, West Sussex, U.K.

Abstract

The relationship of isometric force to sarcomere length transforms, in the intact heart, to the relationship between left ventricular isovolumic pressure and volume. The assumption that this latter relationship is straight and represents an elastance, E_{max}, implies the visco-elastic model which was disproved for muscle in general by Fenn. If the force–length curve is straight, no resulting pressure–volume curve will be convex to the pressure axis due to geometry. There are also data to show that the pressure–volume relationship is non-linear, thus invalidating E_{max}. The uniqueness of the pressure–volume diagram as a unique descriptor of left ventricular mechanical function would be invalidated if the slow response of force to length change proved to be present in the intact heart; present data on that point is contradictory between different laboratories. As long as contractility is normal and systole of sufficient duration, the end-systolic pressure–volume curve is identical to the isovolumic one. Then an increase in end-diastolic volume results in an identical increase in stroke volume (at the same ejection pressure) and end-systolic volume is constant. A shift to the left of the end-systolic pressure–volume curve indicates increased myocardial contractility. A shift to the right indicates either a negative inotropic effect or an abbreviation of systole.

Introduction

Contraction of muscle is best characterized by the relationship between sarcomere length and tension developed at a series of constant sarcomere lengths – the sarcomere length–tension relation – see Chapters 1, 2, and 6. In the intact heart, sarcomere length cannot be controlled. The best we can do is study isovolumic contractions.[1] Left ventricular volume is directly related

H.E.D.J. ter Keurs and M.I.M. Noble (eds), *Starling's Law of the Heart Revisited*. ISBN 978-94-010-7084-3
© 1988, Kluwer Academic Publishers, Dordrecht

to muscle fiber length and pressure to tension. In the ejecting heart, there are a number of output variables which are related to the initial fiber length or end-diastolic volume.[2,3] However, these are different phenomena. A comparable relationship to the isovolumic pressure–volume curve is given by the end-systolic pressure–volume relationship.[4] However, for this to be a unique description of the contractile state, it must be invariant in the face of changes in end-diastolic volume, time, and arterial pressure. A number of studies have challenged this supposition.

The isovolumic pressure–volume curve – relationship to wall tension and fiber length

The relationship between the pressure in the left ventricular cavity and the force developed by the muscle fibers in the ventricular wall is determined by the Laplace law in one form or another. This last phrase covers many possibilities which have led to a rather large literature on the subject. At one end of the spectrum are papers which use oversimplifying assumptions about the shape and form of the ventricle, e.g., that the ventricle is like a thin walled sphere; at the other end of the geometry of the ventricle so that they end up with models of great complexity which can only be handled with large computers. The first approach is too inaccurate to be of use; the second is too complex to be practical. I will quote only one paper which presents what is, in my opinion, the best compromise, but see Chapters 8 and 9 for alternative points of view.

Hefner et al.[5] made no assumptions about shape of wall thickness, but simply considered the situation if the left ventricle (in the imagination) were to be cut through its equator into two hemispheres (Fig. 1). The total force tending to pull the two halves of the ventricle apart (F) would then be equal to the left ventricular cavity pressure (P) multiplied by the cross-sectional area of the cut-across cavity (a):

$$F = Pa \tag{1}$$

The force exerted by the fibers in the wall can then be expressed by dividing F by the total area of the cut-across ventricular wall; this is the equatorial wall stress. From this equation, it can be seen that left ventricular pressure is directly related to force and inversely related to heart size:

$$P = F/a \tag{2}$$

If we assume that cavity cross-sectional area is roughly equal times the square of the radius (r), then:

$$P = F/r^2 \tag{3}$$

This implies that pressure is directly related to force and inversely related to the square of ventricular dimensions.

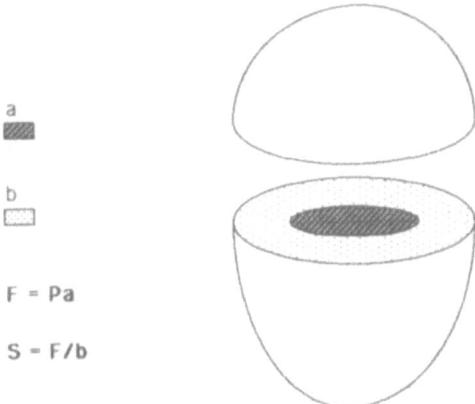

Fig. 1. Hefner's application of the LaPlace Law to the left ventricle. The force tending to pull the two hemispheres apart is the product of pressure and cavity cross)sectional area (Pa). The stress of the myocardial fibers in the meridional direction is this force divided by the "cut" area of muscle, b.

The relationship between volume and ventricular dimensions is as subject to the geometric model assumed as the pressure/force problem. For accurate volume measurement, a complex model such as multiple elliptical cylinders[6] is best. However, in order to relate pressure–volume diagrams to force–length diagrams, it is important to decide whether ventricular filling is of a "1D", "2D" or "3D" type (Fig. 2). The opinion expressed at the Ciba Foundation meeting on Starling's Law[7] is, I think, still valid. It was that the isovolumic contraction and relaxation periods were times when major shape changes occurred, dominated by length changes of the longitudinal fibers. During filling and ejection, volume change occurred in a "2D" fashion. Volume is

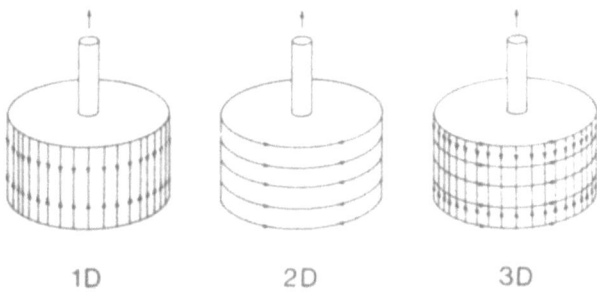

Fig. 2. Simplified concepts of left ventricular geometric changes. A '1D' ventricle would show longitudinal length changes only and perhaps this is the dominant type of change during isovolumic periods of the cardiac cycle. A '2D' ventricle would show circumferential length changes only and perhaps this is the dominant type of change during ejection and filling. Even if longitudinal and circumferential length changes do not occur simultaneously ('3D'), the sequential 1D and 2D changes during the cardiac cycle would mean that the volume changes to be considered in the pressure–volume curve are likely to have a net effect equivalent to 3D.

proportional to r^2 times ventricular length. It is clear from this that volume must increase proportionately much more than fiber length, by a square or even a cube function, while pressure must increase proportionately much less than force because it also depends inversely on heart size.

From this, we can predict with certainty (based on purely geometric considerations) that a straight isometric force-length curve of cardiac muscle will be transformed in a ventricle into an isovolumic pressure–volume curve which is convex to the pressure axis.

Is the isovolumic pressure–volume curve straight? – non-validity of the E_{max} concept

The question of linearity of the pressure–volume relationship requires to be debated because Suga and Sugawa have tried to establish the slope of such a straight line as an index of contractility.[8,9] They call the slope E_{max} to indicate a maximum elastance, assuming that the ventricle behaves like a time varying elastance. This assumption really takes the thinking about cardiac muscle back to the visco-elastic model of Blix[10] (the model Starling had in mind when he likened heart function to "the law of muscle in general"); this theory was disproved by Fenn who found extra heat liberation above that liberated during an isometric contraction when muscle shortened. As Elzinga[11] has recently pointed out, the existence of the Fenn effect,[12] even if not demonstrable in cardiac muscle,[13] must force us to abandon the visco-elastic model for the heart unless we are prepared to propose a completely different mechanism of contraction in heart compared to skeletal muscle. I for one am unequivocably opposed to such a course and cannot accept E or E_{max} of Suga and Sagawa as a real basis for any fundamental concept of contractility.

If this philosophical argument is not convincing, we can equally well reject the E_{max} concept on the pragmatic basis that the pressure–volume curve is certainly not always linear. It is difficult to know which of the curves relating force to sarcomere length (see Chapters 1 and 6) applies to the normal intact situation. At low external calcium ion concentration, the curves are concave to the force axis, at higher activation there is a straight relationship and at even higher calcium concentration the curves are convex to the force axis. These shapes cannot be applied directly to intact heart pressure–volume relationships because the corresponding level of activation is unknown, depending on the internal calcium ion release, and the geometric distortion. However, as discussed in the previous section, a straight force/length relationship must result in a curved pressure–volume relation convex to the pressure axis. A straight pressure–volume relation can only result from a

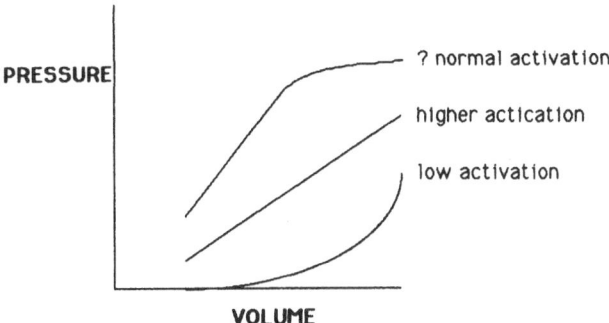

Fig. 3. The effect of increasing contractile state on the isovolumic pressure–volume curve. The straight line case (labeled "higher activation") may not be representative of the normal full contractility which may rather be characterized by a higher convex curve.

concave, low activation force/length curve transformed by the appropriate geometric factors, i.e., there is nothing intrinsically linear about the pressure–volume relationship; it can only be straight by chance. This is not only confirmed by the finding that different laboratories obtain convex curves (e.g. my own) but by the data presented at recent meetings by Burkhoff and Sagawa (see Chapter 8) which I have tried to present schematically in Fig. 3. They ingeniously altered the level of activation by pacing the heart with alternate short and long intervals. The short intervals produced underactivated beats (incomplete mechanical restitution) and the long intervals produced overactivated beats (post-extrasystolic potentiation). The pressure-volume curves of the underactivated beats were concave to the pressure axis, the control curves were straight and the pressure–volume relationship of post-extrasystolic beats was convex to the pressure axis. This family of curves (Fig. 3) is remarkably similar to that found for force/sarcomere length relations in isolated cardiac muscle (see Chapters 1 and 6).

These results prove unequivocally that the pressure–volume relationship is not intrinsically straight and is indeed curved in one way or another. In these circumstances, the universal straight line assumption implied by Emax is untenable. An important reason for not using E_{max} in even a pragmatic way is that it is dangerous from the point of view of misuse in application. For instance, I have come across clinical studies where the authors have determined only two end-systolic pressure/volume data points which were then joined with a straight line. It must be obvious from the discussion in this section that such procedures are very likely to result in erroneous conclusions. From this point of view, I think it would be more healthy for E_{max} to be abandoned altogether.

Does the isovolumic pressure–volume curve change with time following a volume change? – relationship to the slow phase of tension development

When the length of isolated cardiac muscle is increased, there is an immediate increase in developed force, followed by a slower rise in contractility over a time course of several minutes. It is possible to estimate the amount of calcium released intracellularly (i.e. activation) by injecting the bioluminescent protein aequorin, which emits light in the presence of free calcium ions; the amount of light can be measured and calibrated to give reasonable quantification of the "calcium transient" that occurs following each stimulus (see Chapter 3). The immediate force increment upon lengthening the muscle is not accompanied by any change in calcium transient. This implies some other mechanism than altered calcium release to explain the force/length curve. It will be seen in Chapter 1 that there is evidence that the mechanism is a length induced change in the sensitivity of the contractile proteins for calcium. The more slowly developing increase in force is accompanied by an increase in the light signal indicating that the mechanism of this component is an increase in activation (increased internal calcium ion release). These observations[14] are of great importance because there was previously confusion as to whether the length induced increase in force was fundamentally different from an increase in contractility.[15] We now know that this is indeed true for the immediate length induced force increase but that the slow component is indistinguishable in mechanism (at the moment) from a contractility increase produced by an intervention such as post-extrasystolic potentiation.

A study by Tucci et al.[16] apparently confirmed that the same immediate and slow components were present in the response of left ventricular isovolumic pressure to an increase in volume. If this observation is correct, it has serious implications for the use of the pressure–volume diagram as a definition of contractile state. The studies of Frank[1] through to the modern ones of Hefner[17] and Sagawa[18] all point to the pressure–volume diagram as the "absolute" and "unique" description of the contractility of the heart. Changes in volume are supposed to move pressure up the curve only. But if Tucci et al.'s observation is correct, all of that is wrong because, during the slow component of pressure response to volume, there is a slow drift of the entire pressure–volume relationship to the left (Fig. 4). In other words, as soon as one tries to move up a given pressure–volume line there is a slow positive inotropic effect moving the line upwards, due to increased internal calcium release. If this is really true the entire concept of the pressure–volume curve would have to be abandoned and there would no longer be any hope of distinguishing volume induced effects from changes in contractility. My own opinion, based on present experiments (partly indicated in a preliminary

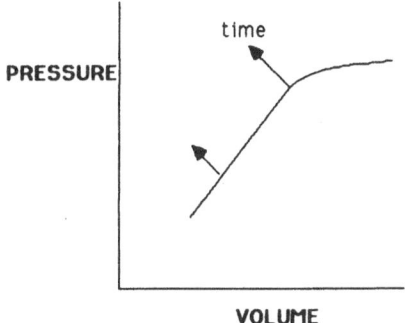

Fig. 4. The effect on the pressure–volume curve of the slow component of the contractile response to increased sarcomere and fiber length.

abstract[19]) is that the slow component is not present to a significant extent in the intact heart. It will be necessary for us to complete these studies and publish them, and for the ensuing debate over the different results from different laboratories to reach a generally accepted conclusion, before we will know whether to scrap the conventional view or not. I am in the unusual position of representing the view that the conventional analysis of cardiac mechanics, in terms of the pressure–volume relationship as a cardinal functional descriptor, will be vindicated. However, until that time I must point out that it is under a cloud.

Is the end-systolic pressure–volume curve identical with the isovolumic pressure–volume curve?

Up to this point I have dealt only with the pressure–volume diagram defined by isovolumic contractions. In the ejecting heart, the isovolumic contraction period is followed by ejection, i.e., decreasing volume at systolic left ventricular pressure. When this is plotted in the diagram, ejection appears as a horizontal segment to the left (Fig. 5a); the pressure at which ejection occurs is well below the pressure that would have been attained isovolumically. Ejection is shown to continue in Fig. 5a until volume reaches the pressure-volume line; further ejections at higher left ventricular pressure (Fig. 5b) enable further points on the pressure–volume curve to be reached at each end-systole. That this often happens is well illustrated by Janicki, Weber, Janicki and Hefner.[217] On the basis of their experiment,, these authors therefore proposed that the end-systolic pressure–volume relationship was identical to the isovolumic one. Contractility in the ejecting heart could therefore be defined by the same pressure–volume relationship as the isovolumic heart by making the necessary measurements at end-systole.

130

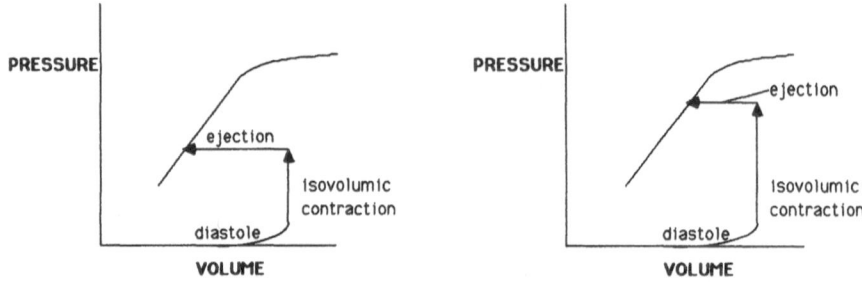

Fig. 5. Determination of the end)systolic pressure volume relationship in ejecting hearts. The heart ejects down at any given ejection pressure to the volume on the isovolumic pressure–volume curve from which that pressure would have been developed isovolumically. Ejection at one pressure determines only one point on the curve. In order to determine the whole curve, ejections must be studied at many pressures of which two are illustrated schematically in panels a and b.

This important contention has been seriously challenged. In the first place, if one does the comparable experiment with force and muscle length in isolated papillary muscle, it is usual to find (certainly in my experience) that the end-systolic force–length relationship is to the right of the isometric curve. It has further been shown in intact heart studies of a number of authors including those of Sagawa's group that the end-systolic pressure-volume relationship is to the right of the isovolumic curve (Fig. 6). One may well therefore assert that if the end-systolic pressure–volume curve is not always the same as the isovolumic one, the concept of a unique pressure–volume diagram as a definition of contractility is untenable.

I reject this view and again (uncharacteristically for me) defend the conventional concept. The main problem with pressure–volume diagrams is that they remove the important dimension of time. On examining those experiments in which volume did not reach the isovolumic pressure–volume line at end-systole, it was always because ejection was of insufficient duration

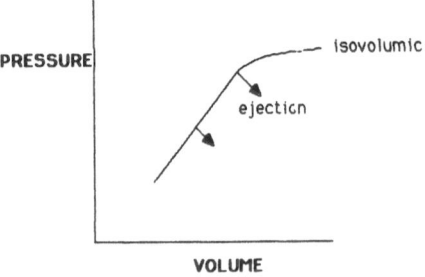

Fig. 6. Pressure–volume curves determined at end-systole by the method illustrated in Fig. 5 are reported sometimes to lie to the right of the curve determined isovolumically in the same heart (arrows). Reasons for this are discussed in the text.

for volume to have time to reach end-point. One such condition is under circumstances of depressed muscle contraction which is sometimes due to problems with the preparation. In depressed myocardium, the velocity of shortening is reduced so that more time than normal is required during ejection for the volume to reduce to the predicted end-systolic value; this problem is compounded by the fact that depressed myocardium sometimes has an abbreviated systole as well. Abbreviation of systole is the reason for the non-superposition of isovolumic and end-systolic pressure–volume curves sometimes encountered with catecholamine stimulation. I also think it could explain the effects encountered when the piston controlling volume in Sagawa's preparation is made to simulate different impedances.[20] In my opinion one may state that the two relationships do superimpose as long as the duration of systole is adequately maintained and not interrupted by premature relaxation.

A consequence of the identity of the isovolumic and end-systolic curves is that in ejecting hearts at a given ejection pressure, an increase in end-diastolic volume will result in an identical absolute increment in stroke volume. This is illustrated in Fig. 7, in which a control pressure–volume path is illustrated in panel A. The length of the arrow marked "ejection" represents the stroke volume (i.e., change of volume during ejection.) When ejection starts from a higher end-diastolic volume (panel B) the increase in length of the ejection arrow is identical to the increment on the volume axis of end-diastolic volume. A characteristic of hearts in which the end-systolic pressure) + volume line is to the right of the isovolumic one (Fig. 6) is that the deviation to the right becomes greater as the heart is distended more, i.e., the increment in stroke volume is less than the increment in end-diastolic volume. If, however, the end-systolic and isovolumic curves superimpose, as I contend they do if contractility is normal, a plot of stroke volume against end-diastolic volume must have a positive slope of one and an increase in end-diastolic volume is associated with a constant end-systolic volume. I have found that measurement of left ventricular cavity volume in intact animals is very difficult but I think I succeeded many years ago using implanted tantalum markers to outline the cavity and biplane X-ray cinefluorimetry to record their position in two planes.[21] I altered end-diastolic volume by changing the filling time (having established that the positive and negative effects of that intervention cancel out in the intact animal to give a flat force–frequency relationship.[6,22] Under these experimental conditions, the absolute changes in stroke volume and end-diastolic volume were indeed not statistically different and end-systolic volume was constant.[6] I therefore interpret those old experiments as confirming that in the normal, conscious dog, the end-systolic pressure–volume relationship is constant for a given inotropic state.

132

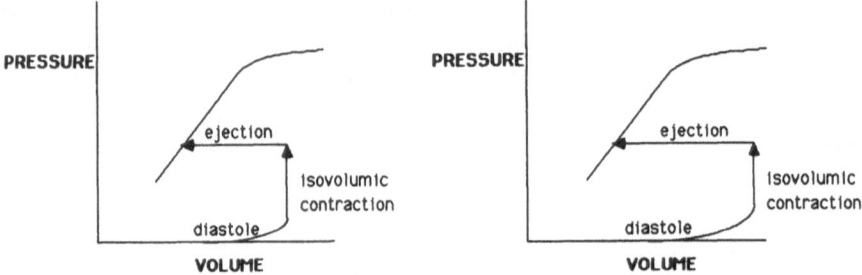

Fig. 7. The course followed by pressure and volume in ejecting hearts (at a given ejection pressure) from a control end-diastolic volume (a) and an increased end-diastolic volume (b).

Why should the ventricle contract down (given sufficient time) to the volume from which it would develop end-systolic pressure isovolumically At that volume the ventricle is at the volume at which it can maintain the applied pressure isovolumically but is unable to contract down against that pressure. Similarly the sarcomeres in the ventricular wall are at the length where they can just maintain the prevailing force isometrically but at which they are unable to shorten against that load. If one were able to prolong the activation of the muscle at exactly the same level, the muscle would remain in contracture at that same length and developed force until relaxation was eventually allowed. This is not so obvious in skeletal muscle which often works on a descending limb of its force/length curve. Cardiac muscle has no such descending limb and the normal heart has no descending limb to its pressure-volume curve.[23]

Interpretation of changes in position of the pressure–volume curve

With an isovolumically determined curve, an increase in contractility or positive inotropic effect causes a leftward shift of the curve, i.e., for any given ventricular volume an increase in contractility is manifest by an increase in developed isovolumic pressure. With a decrease in contractility or negative inotropic effect, the opposite is true; there is a rightward shift of the curve and less isovolumic pressure is developed at any given volume.

When considering the curve determined at end-systole in ejecting hearts, the same holds true as above for positive inotropic effects provided that activation time is maintained. A rightward shift occurs either as a result of a negative inotropic effect, or a reduction in velocity of shortening (which is in any case a manifestation of a negative inotropic effect), or a shortening of the duration of activation.

Is the isovolumic pressure–volume curve valid in the light of the Anrep effect

The nomenclature of this subject is confusing. Anrep studied supposed inotropic effects of changes in arterial pressure and filling. it is much more satisfactory to separate these two influences which have different mechanisms. The inotropic effect of a change in filling is the slow component of the response of developed pressure to a change of volume. This has already been discussed at length above. Sarnoff[24] regarded the Anrep effect solely as a positive inotropic response to an increase of aortic pressure which he regarded as a manifestation of homeometric autoregulation. However, he included the Bowditch effect in homeometric autoregulation; since the Bowditch effect is another completely different mechanism, this is also unsatisfactory. Moreover, an increase in ejection load can also cause a negative inotropic effect.[25] In the best study of these effects, Donald et al.[26] called the positive inotropic effect "homeometric autoregulation" and the negative inotropic effect "anti-homeometric autoregulation"! There is an element of absurdity in this nomenclature because this is a length independent (i.e. homeometric) negative inotropic effect. I think it would be preferable to call these responses "the positive and negative effects of increased load".

These effects, if present, would invalidate the end-systolic pressure–volume relationship as a unique descriptor of the contractile state of the heart because as one increased aortic pressure to delineate the curve (Fig. 5), the contractile state would change.[30] Thus if there was a positive inotropic effect of increased load (the Anrep effect in Sarnoff's meaning), the pressure–volume curve would be shifting to the left (Fig. 8) as it was being measured. The study of Donald et al.[27] showed that whether one obtained a positive or negative inotropic effect of increased load in an isolated papillary muscle depended on the temperature and stimulation frequency. They defined a

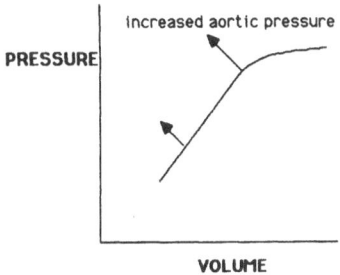

Fig. 8. The effect on the end-systolic pressure–volume diagram if the heart has a positive inotropic response to increased systolic load.

temperature/frequency isopleth defining the combinations of these variables which resulted in neither effect. The temperature and normal resting heart rate of the intact heart in situ lies on this isopleth, indicating that neither effect need be expected. We studied this question in the intact dog in some detail.[27] We used the maximum rate of rise of left ventricular pressure as a measure of contractility (for justification –) see below) and were unable to detect any significant inotropic effect of raising aortic pressure. We also reviewed the entire literature on this subject. In my opinion therefore, in the normal heart, the positive and negative inotropic effects of increased load are not of sufficient magnitude to invalidate the use of the end-systolic pressure–volume curve.

What about "ventricular function curves", the relationship of stroke volume and work to end-diastolic volume, and Starling's "Law"?

Starling measured the output of the isolated heart-lung preparation ejecting against a "waterfall" type aortic resistor, and found that this variable increased with right atrial pressure and then decreased. Elzinga has recently given a thoughtful and detailed analysis of how Starling's thoughts progressed from these findings.[11] Starling was struck by the similar rise and fall with muscle length of (a) skeletal muscle isometric force, (b) skeletal muscle heat liberation and (c) his cardiac output against a fixed pressure. He therefore thought that all three of these variables were measures of the "energy output" of the muscle. Therefore he proposed that the "energy output however measured" was a function of the initial length of the cardiac muscle fibers and that this made the heart follow the "law of muscle in general".[28] Since he was thinking of the viscoelastic model of Blix[10] which was disproved by Fenn,[12] he was wrong about the law of muscle. Therefore his own concept of heart function can hardly be considered to be a "law". But he was also wrong to think that cardiac output was an equivalent measure to isometric force on the energy output of the heart.

This can easily be appreciated from examination of the pressure–volume ejection loops at constant aortic pressure within the pressure–volume diagram (Fig. 7). It can be appreciated that from every end-diastolic volume the heart ejects down to the same end-diastolic volume, i.e. the heart only operates at one single point on the pressure–volume (and muscle force–length) curve. Measurements of stroke volume (or cardiac output = stroke volume X heart rate) or stroke work (= stroke volume X pressure) plotted against end-diastolic volume (or any pressure related to end-diastolic, "filling" pressure) give no information whatever about the position or shape of the pressure-volume curve or the length–tension curve of the muscle comprising the left ventricular wall. Therefore it is quite wrong to think that energy output measured in any way can be plotted against an index of heart size to yield a "ventricular function curve". One must state specifically that isovolumic pressure development is a function of the initial length of the muscle fibers.

A further word of caution is necessary about the use of stroke work, which is a function of aortic pressure. Therefore its use is only interpretable if the aortic pressure is constant. But then the changes in stroke work are identical to the changes in stroke volume, so one might as well plot stroke volume anyway. When end-diastolic pressure (or related pressure) is used instead of volume considerable distortion of the relationship occurs.[29]

How are other variables measurable in ejecting hearts related to end-diastolic volume?

There is a large and contentious literature on the validity or otherwise of various "indices of contractility" which I will make no attempt to review here. My own position has been made clear.[31] It can be summarized by saying that none of these indices have any intrinsic validity like that of the pressure-volume diagram. Some of them may have practical validity if found to be insensitive to changes in end-diastolic volume and aortic pressure. I have consistently thought that two of these indices are likely to be valid in some circumstances:

(1) The maximum rate of rise of left ventricular pressure (LVdP/dtmax). This is an isovolumic event as long as it occurs before aortic valve opening. Under those circumstances, changes in aortic pressure have no effect. It is obtained by differentiating equation (1):

$$dF/dt = (a)dP/dt + (P)da/dt \qquad (1)$$

If we assume that isovolumic contraction is isometric, the rate of change of left ventricular cavity cross-sectional area, da/dt, will be zero because the area is then constant. Thus:

$$dP/dt = (dF/dt)/a$$

This means that dP/dt is directly related to the rate of rise of force in the wall of the heart and inversely related to the cavity area. Therefore when end-diastolic volume is increased, the consequent rise in dF/dt tends to cause dP/dt to increase, but the rise in cavity cross-sectional area itself causes dP/dt to decrease. The final result depends on the balance between these two effects and that balance may be, and sometimes is, no change in LVdP/dtmax. Each preparation must be tested to check on this before the index is used as an index of contractility.

(2) The maximum rate of rise of left ventricular outflow, maximum acceleration. In the conscious dog, this index also turns out to be rather insensitive to changes in end-diastolic volume[31] and I have suggested that this could be because the increased force doing the accelerating is balanced by the increased mass of blood to be accelerated. The index is inferior to LVdP/dt-max in that it is affected by changes in aortic pressure, particularly increases in pressure. However, it is less sensitive to aortic pressure when the latter is low, so that the index may become more useful under these circumstances when LVdP/dtmax is in danger of becoming non-isovolumic. However, one must once again stress that as a pragmatic index only; maximum acceleration must be tested in each preparation to which it is applied. For instance, I have found that maximum acceleration is very much more affected by changes in end-diastolic volume in man than in dog. Even so, in man it has the great advantage of being measureable non-invasively by transcutaneous Doppler techniques.

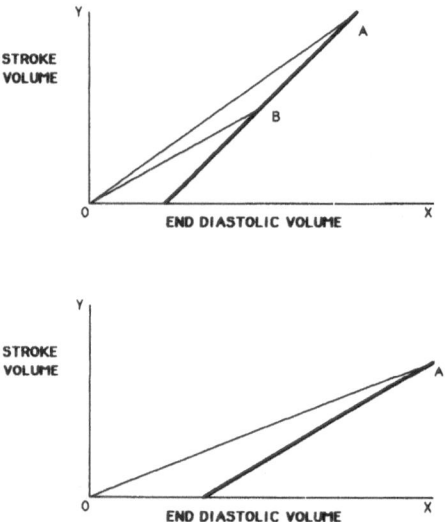

Fig. 9. a. In the normal heart with an end-diastolic pressure–volume curve which is independent of end-diastolic volume (i.e. constant end-systolic volume for a given pressure), the relationship between stroke volume and end-diastolic volume for a given systolic pressure is illustrated by the bold line, with a slope of 1.0. The intercept on the end-diastolic volume axis is the constant end-systolic volume. The ejection fraction at point B is the tangent of the angle BOX, and increases at point A to the tangent of the angle AOX. This increase is proportionately much less than the corresponding % increase in stroke volume (= % increase in stroke work = % increase in cardiac output (if heart rate constant) from B to A. b. In a depressed or diseased heart the end-systolic volume increases and the slope of the relationship between stroke volume and end-diastolic volume may be less than 1.0. The ejection fraction at point A would now be the lower tangent of the angle AOX in panel b, accurately reflecting the deterioration in mechanical performance compared to panel a.

A note should be added about the popular clinical index called ejection fraction, i.e. (stroke volume)/(end-diastolic volume). As discussed above, the relationship between stroke volume and end-diastolic volume in the normal heart is a straight line with a slope of 1.0 (Fig. 9a). There is an intercept on the end-diastolic volume axis which has the same value as the (constant) end-systolic volume. All this follows from study of the pressure–volume diagram as long as the aortic pressure remains constant (e.g., normotensive patients). The ejection fraction is the tangent of the angle subtended at the origin by any particular point on the line under consideration (Fig. 9a). It can be appreciated from the figure that this angle increases with increasing end-diastolic volume but not so much as stroke volume, i.e. there is less sensitivity of this index to changes in end-diastolic volume than is the case with other ejection variables. Indeed, in man I have found it less sensitive to changes in end-diastolic volume than maximum acceleration. When one carries out all clinical measurements with the subject in the same posture, filling differences are minimized. If the pressure–volume diagram of the patient is moved to the right and the end) systolic volume is increased due to myocardial depression, the resulting stroke volume/end-diastolic volume diagram will have a larger intercept (Fig. 9b). The decrease in the angle subtended at the origin can be seen in the figure. Thus, ejection fraction is quite a good pragmatic index of the pressure-volume status of the normotensive patient; its popularity amongst clinicians is justified.

Why the terms "preload" and "afterload" should be expunged from the heart literature

In the early days of isolated muscle experimentation, apparatus for controlling the length and/or sarcomere length were lacking. Therefore physiologists applied a little tension to the resting muscle to set the starting conditions. This was done by hanging a weight on the end of the vertically oriented muscle – the preload. This practice has now been abandoned because with an electromagnetic lever, one can now set the resting sarcomere length monitored optically. Sarcomere length is the variable which determines the contractile performance of the muscle according to the force/sarcomere length relationship (see above). Even if preloads were still used in isolated muscle experiments, there is nothing comparable to them in intact heart experiments. The nearest equivalent to preload in the intact heart would be the end-diastolic left ventricular wall stress; it does at least have the same dimensions. Hardly anybody even tries to measure this. The word preload is loosely applied to all sorts of variables which certainly do not have the same or equivalent physical or physiological meaning and all have different dimensions. Since all these variables have their own accurate definitions, they should be called by their proper names so that everybody knows what is being measured. For instance, to call pulmonary wedge pressure "preload" instead of its own name is silly, inaccurate and confusing.

Similar arguments apply to afterload, a weight that the muscle lifted during contraction in the old-fashioned apparatus. The muscle lifted exactly the same weight during the whole of the shortening period. This *never* happens in the intact heart because, as must follow from equation (1), the left ventricular wall stress falls off drastically during the ejection period. To apply the word "afterload" to any other variable obscures proper understanding. I am often rebuked for these views by people who use the terms preload and afterload in the intact animal or patient. They say "We use these terms because everybody then knows what we mean". When I then interrogate them to find out what *they* mean, they usually do not know. The conclusion seems to me overwhelming that the general use of these terms is an example of the worst sort of jargon.

Conclusion

The pressure–volume analysis presented in this Chapter should provide a framework for understanding most of intact heart mechanics in terms which are unambiguous. The only factor lacking in the pressure–volume analysis as a framework is the important dimension of time.

References

1. Frank O (1985). Zur Dynamik des Herzmuskels. Zeitschrift faar Biologie 32: 370–447, translated by Chapman CB and Wasserman E (1959). Am Heart J 58: 282–317, 467–478.
2. Patterson SW, Piper H and Starling EH (1914). The regulation of the heart beat. J Physiol 8: 465–513.
3. Patterson WS and Starling EH (1914). On the mechanical factors which determine the output of the ventricles. J Physiol 48: 357–379.
4. Sagawa K (1981). Editorial. The end-systolic pressure–volume relation of the ventricle: Definition, modifications and clinical use. Circulation 63: 1223–1227.
5. Hefner LL, Sheffield LT, Cobbs GC and Klip W (1962). Relation between mural force and pressure in the left ventricle of the dog. Circ Res 811: 654–663.
6. Noble MIM, Wyler J, Milne ENC, Trenchard D and Guz A (1969). Effect of changes in heart rate on left ventricular performance in conscious dogs. Circ Res 24: 285–295.
7. Ciba Foundation Symposium (1974). The Physiological Basis of Starling's Law of the Heart. Elsevier:Excerpta Medica:North Holland, Amsterdam.
8. Suga H and Sagawa K (1974). Instantaneous pressure–volume relationships and their ratio in the excised supported canine left ventricle. Circ Res 35: 117–126.
9. Sagawa K, Suga H, Shoukas A and Bakalar K (1977). End-systolic pressure/volume ratio: a new index of ventricular contractility. Am J Cardiol 40: 748–753.

10. Blix M (1982). Die Lange und die Spannung des Muskels. Skand Arch Physiol 3: 295–318.
11. Elzinga G (1986). Cardiac pump functions; what would Starling say Proceedings of the IUPS 16: L354.01.
12. Fenn WO (1923). A quantitative comparison between the energy liberated and the work performed by the isolated sartorius muscle of the frog. J Physiol 58: 175–203.
13. Gibbs CL, Mommaerts WFHM and Ricchiuti NV (1967). Energetics of cardiac contractions. J Physiol 191: 25–46.
14. Allen DG and Kurihara S (1982). The effects of muscle length on intracellular calcium transients in mammalian cardiac muscle. J Physiol 273: 597–615.
15. Jewell BR (1977). A re-examination of the influence of muscle length on myocardial performance. Circ Res 40: 221–230.
16. Tucci PJF, Bregagnollo EA, Spadaro J, Cicogna AC and Ribiero MCL (1984). Length dependent activation studied in the isovolumic blood-perfused dog heart. Circ Res: 5559–66.
17. Weber KT, Janicki JS and Hefner LL (1976). Left ventricular force–length relations of isovolumic and ejecting contractions. Am J Physiol 231: 337–343.
18. Sagawa K (1978). The ventricular pressure–volume diagram revisited. Circ Res 43: 677–687.
19. Pettersson K, Drake-Holland AJ and Noble MIM (1985). Isometric contractions in the isovolumically beating dog heart. Cardiovasc Res 19: 521.
20. Maughan WL, Sunagawa K, Burkhoff D and Sagawa K (1984). Effect of arterial impedence changes on the end-systolic pressure–volume relation. Circ Res 54: 595–602.
21. Noble MIM, Milne ENC, Goerke RJ, Carlsson E, Domenech RJ, Saunders KB and Hoffman JIE (1969a). Left ventricular filling and diastolic pressure–volume relations in the conscious dog. Circ Res 24: 269–283.
22. Pidgeon J, Lab M, Elzinga G, Papadoyannis D and Noble MIM (1980). The contractile state of cat and dog heart in relation to the interval between beats. Circ Res 47: 559–567.
23. Monroe RG, Gamble WJ, LaFarge CG, Kumar AE and Manasek FJ (1970). Left ventricular performance at high end-diastolic pressures in isolated perfused dog hearts. Circ Res 26: 85–100.
24. Sarnoff SJ and Mitchell JH (1962). The control of the function of the heart. Handbook of Physiology, section 2 Circulation, vol 1, 489–532. American Physiological Society, Washington DC.
25. Parmley WW, Brutsaert DL and Sonnenblick (1969). Effects of altered loading on contractile events in isolated cat papillary muscle. Circ Res 24: 521–532.
26. Donald TC, Peterson DM, Walker AA and Hefner LL 91976). Afterload-induced homeometric autoregulation in isolated cardiac muscle. Am J Physiol 231: 545–550.
27. Elzinga G, Noble MIM and Stubbs J (1977). The effect of an increase in aortic pressure upon the inotropic state of cat and dog left ventricles. J Physiol 273: 597–615.
28. Starling EH (1918). The Linacre Lecture on the Law of the Heart, Longmans, Green & Co, London.
29. Noble MIM (1978). The Frank-Starling curve. Clinical Science 54: 1–7.
30. Bos GC van den, Elzinga G, Westerhoff N and Noble MIM (1973). Problems in the use of indices of myocardial contractility. Cardiovasc Res 7: 834–848.
31. Noble MIM, Trenchard D and Guz A (1966). Left ventricular ejection in conscious dogs. I. Measurement and significance of the maximum acceleration of blood from the left ventricle. Circ Res 19: 139–147

Index

DEVELOPMENTS IN CARDIOVASCULAR MEDICINE

Recent volumes

Lowell Stone, H., Weglicki, W.B., eds.: Pathology of cardiovascular injury. 1985. ISBN 0-89838-743-4.

Meyer, J., Erbel, R., Rupprecht, H.J., eds.: Improvement of myocardial perfusion. 1985. ISBN 0-89838-748-5.

Reiber, J.H.C., Serruys, P.W., Slager, C.J.: Quantitative coronary and left ventricular cineangiography. 1986. ISBN 0-89838-760-4.

Fagard, R.H., Bekaert, I.E., eds.: Sports cardiology. 1986. ISBN 0-89838-782-5.

Reiber, J.H.C., Serruys, P.W., eds.: State of the art in quantitative coronary arteriography. 1986. ISBN 0-89838-804-X.

Roelandt, J., ed.: Color Doppler Flow Imaging. 1986. ISBN 0-89838-806-6.

Van der Wall, E.E., ed.: Noninvasive imaging of cardiac metabolism. 1986. ISBN 0-89838-812-0.

Liebman, J., Plonsey, R., Rudy, Y., eds.: Pediatric and fundamental electrocardiography. 1986. ISBN 0-89838-815-5.

Hilger, H.H., Hombach, V., Rashkind, W.J., eds.: Invasive cardiovascular therapy. 1987. ISBN 0-89838-818-X

Serruys, P.W., Meester, G.T., eds.: Coronary angioplasty: a controlled model for ischemia. 1986. ISBN 0-89838-819-8.

Tooke, J.E., Smaje, L.H.: Clinical investigation of the microcirculation. 1986. ISBN 0-89838-819-8.

Van Dam, R.Th., Van Oosterom, A., eds.: Electrocardiographic body surface mapping. 1986. ISBN 0-89838-834-1.

Spencer, M.P., ed.: Ultrasonic diagnosis of cerebrovascular disease. 1987. ISBN 0-89838-836-8.

Legato, M.J., ed.: The stressed heart. 1987. ISBN 0-89838-849-X.

Safar, M.E., ed.: Arterial and venow systems in essential hypertension. 1987. ISBN 0-89838-857-0.

Roelandt, J., ed.: Digital techniques in echocardiography. 1987. ISBN 0-89838-861-9.

Dhalla, N.S. et al., eds.: Pathophysiology of heart disease. 1987. ISBN 0-89838-864-3.

Dhalla, N.S. et al., eds.: Heart function and metabolism. 1987. ISBN 0-89838-865-1.

Dhalla, N.S. et al., eds.: Myocardial Ischemia. 1987. ISBN 0-89838-866-X.

Beamish, R.E. et al., eds.: Pharmacological aspects of heart disease. 1987. ISBN 0-89838-867-8.

Ter Keurs, H.E.D.J., Tyberg, J.V., eds.: Mechanics of the circulation. 1987. ISBN 0-89838-870-8

Sideman, S., Beyar, R., eds.: Activation, metabolism and perfusion of the heart. 1987. ISBN 0-89838-871-6.

Aliot, E., Lazzara, R., eds.: Ventricular tachycardias. 1987. ISBN 0-89838-881-3.

Schneeweiss, A. et al., eds.: Cardiovascular drug therapy in the elderly. 1987. ISBN 0-89838-883-X.

Chapman, J.V., Sgalambro, A., eds.: Basic concepts in Doppler echocardiography. 1987. ISBN 0-89838-888-0

Chien, S. et al., eds.: Clinical hemocheology. 1987. ISBN 0-89838-807-4.

Morganroth, J., ed.: Congestive heart failure. 1987. ISBN 0-89838-955-0.

Messerli, F.H., ed.: Cardiovascular disease in the elderly. 2nd ed. 1988. ISBN 0-89838-962-3.

Heintzen, P.H., Bürsch, J.H., eds.: Progress in digital angiocardiography. 1988. ISBN 0-89838-965-8.

Scheinman, M.A., ed.: Catheter ablation of cardiac arrhythmias. 1988. ISBN 0-89838-967-4.

Spaan, J.A.E., Bruschke, A.V.G., Gittenberger-de Groot, A.C., eds.: Coronary circulation. 1987. ISBN 0-89838-978-X.

Visser, C., Kan, G., Meltzer, R., eds.: Echocardiography in coronary artery disease. 1988. ISBN 0-89838-979-8.

Bayés de Luna, A., Betriu, A., Permanyer, G., eds.: Therapeutics in cardiology. 1988. ISBN 0-89838-981-X.

Mirvis, D.M., ed.: Body surface electrocardiographic mapping. 1988. ISBN 0-89838-983-6.

Konstam, M.A., Isner, J.M., eds.: The right ventricle. 1988. ISBN 0-89838-987-9.

Kappagoda, C.T., Greenwood, P.V., eds.: Long-term management of patients after myocardial infarction. 1988. ISBN 0-89838-352-8.

Gaasch, W.H., Levine, H.J., eds.: Chronic aortic regurgitation. 1988. ISBN 0-89838-364-1.

Singal, P.K., ed.: Oxygen radicals in the pathophysiology of heart disease. 1988. ISBN 0-89838-375-7.

Reiber, J.H.C., Serruys, P.W., eds.: New developments in quantitative coronary arteriography. 1988. ISBN 0-89838-377-3.

Morganroth, J., Moore, E.N., eds.: Silent myocardial ischemia. 1988. ISBN 0-89838-380-3.

Ter Keurs, H.E.D.J., Noble, M.I.M., eds.: Starling's law of the heart revisited. 1988. ISBN 0-89838-382-X.

KLUWER ACADEMIC PUBLISHERS
DORDRECHT / BOSTON / LONDON